THE
BURN

THE
BURN

Haylie Pomroy
with Eve Adamson

FOREWORD BY JACQUELINE FIELDS, MD

BANTAM PRESS

LONDON · TORONTO · SYDNEY · AUCKLAND · JOHANNESBURG

TRANSWORLD PUBLISHERS
61–63 Uxbridge Road, London W5 5SA
www.transworldbooks.co.uk

Transworld is part of the Penguin Random House group of companies
whose addresses can be found at global.penguinrandomhouse.com

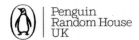

First published in Great Britain in 2015 by Bantam Press
an imprint of Transworld Publishers

A CIP catalogue record for this book is available from the British Library.

ISBN 9780593075036

Typeset in 11/14.5pt Minion Pro
Printed and bound by CPI Group (UK) Ltd, Croydon, CR0 4YY

Penguin Random House is committed to a sustainable future for
our business, our readers and our planet. This book is made
from Forest Stewardship Council® certified paper.

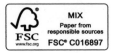

1 3 5 7 9 10 8 6 4 2

How can I title a book *The Burn* and not dedicate it
to my hot husband? Your love has given me the passion
and fuel to ignite my burning desire to help others.

CONTENTS

Barn's burnt down . . . now I can see the moon.

—MASAHIDE, JAPANESE POET (1657–1723)

FOREWORD

I remember the days when Haylie Pomroy was in Colorado a lot more often. That was before she became the diet world sensation that she is now. We all miss those days when we felt like we had her and all her incredible strategies to ourselves. Although Haylie no longer lives in Fort Collins, Colorado, where I run my integrative medicine clinic, The Healing Gardens Health Center, she still comes back to visit us every month or so to see patients. We have come to terms with the fact that we must share Haylie with the world. Her knowledge is too valuable to keep quiet.

Haylie and I have collaborated professionally for more than twenty years, so I consider it an honour and a privilege to write the Foreword for her latest book, *The Burn*. First, Haylie herself is a phenomenon. She has been a part of my life for many years, and my patients love meeting with her. As she has become busier and more sought-after, she hasn't been able to be here as often, so thank goodness she started writing books! Whenever my patients have a weight issue, I refer them to her first book, *The Fast Metabolism Diet*. In fact, it is required reading in my clinic, and almost *all* my patients are now on track to a healthy lifestyle. That's not something a lot of doctors can say because compliance is such a big issue with lifestyle changes. But it is obvious to me—and everyone here—that Haylie's programmes have that special something that keeps people on track. My patients always say that when they read her writing, it feels like she is in the room with them, teaching and inspiring them to get excited about taking charge of their health. Many of my patients who have failed with other weight-loss programmes saw success while on hers.

I am even more excited about this new book. In *The Burn*, Haylie takes her programme to the next level. For those patients who plateau in weight loss, Haylie provides a clear plan and strategy for getting past that stage. The programmes in this book are also excellent for shaking things up, repairing post-indulgence issues, and combatting many different kinds of weight-related metabolic problems. In the book, Haylie clearly describes the three big issues that contribute to stalled weight loss:

- Inflammation
- Digestive issues
- Hormonal imbalance

Then she shows you exactly how to solve them. And guess how she does it? If you know Haylie at all, you know that it will be through food.

Haylie and I have always shared the same focus of care: food is medicine. This book is a fantastic gift, full of wisdom and yummy details showing how food is the answer to continued and sustained weight loss, as well as to the resolution of many chronic problems that plague us, from rashes and bloating to water retention and PMS.

I've been in medicine for more than twenty-five years, and it is clear to me that at least 85 per cent of chronic diseases in this country are due to poor diet and lifestyle choices. Haylie is part of the solution. Her books can truly help transform this cultural problem. Slowing and even reversing chronic disease is about changing diet and lifestyle. I have spent years educating patients on these types of transformations, but Haylie's books can spread this knowledge far and wide. I can only hope all doctors who desire to implement this kind of knowledge in their practices use both Haylie's books, *The Burn* and *The Fast Metabolism Diet*, as valuable resources in their clinics.

Haylie has certainly changed my patients' health and, more specifically, generated a lot of weight loss around here, not to mention the reduction of cardiac risk, diabetes risk, sleep disorders and even depression. So doctors, patients and readers take note! The answers lie within the covers of this book. Health is not a mystery, but if you need a guide, Haylie is here for you. I'm certainly glad that she has been there for me.

—*Jacqueline Fields, MD*

THE
BURN

Introduction:
Welcome to *The Burn*

You're stuck, and I can help.

This is a book for people who need weight loss intervention. It is for people who are stuck and can't get themselves out alone. If you have hit a weight loss plateau, it's as if an invisible barrier were blocking the way to that magical number you long to see on the scale. You are stuck. If you need to lose weight fast and you don't have a year, or six months, or even one month, your goal can feel unattainable. You are stuck. Maybe you need a maximum change in appearance in a minimum amount of time—class reunion? job interview? first date? wedding? beach vacation?—and you have no idea how to do it. You are stuck. Or maybe you need a serious jump-start before making a major lifestyle change, but you don't have any jumper cables. You are stuck.

But you don't have to be.

If you can't lose the weight you need to lose, there is always a reason. Always. Your body is a beautifully complex laboratory of biochemical reactions, and all it takes to get you stuck is for one little thing to go wrong. Maybe it is inflammation and water retention. Maybe it is a digestive problem. Maybe it's your hormones. Whatever it is, it has nothing to do with your willpower. Your body wants to be slim, healthy, strong and energized, and if it's not, then something in the system has gone awry. Something has gotten stuck.

Now you have a problem, and a certain amount of time to fix it. You need to lose weight and look good *fast*. Maybe it's a special event, and you are ready to be amazing. Maybe you need to blow through those last eight pounds to finally reach your goal weight. Maybe your diet isn't working anymore, and you need to get back on the weight loss fast track. Maybe you need to look fabulous by Friday. Maybe you want to depuff your face, get rid of belly bloat, or be sleeker and tighter, from cheekbones to calves. Maybe you've had a health scare such as pre-diabetes or fatty liver disease, and your doctor wants you to kick-start weight loss fast. Or maybe you want to feel better, have more energy, or just feel like yourself again—and you don't want to waste another day.

I've worked with thousands of clients who have lost hundreds of thousands of pounds. Though I've never had the pleasure of meeting some of my virtual clients, we recently tracked a group of individuals on one of my programmes who lost *over 130,000 pounds in less than eight months*. Why does this happen with clients I've never even met, when they don't get my individual attention? Because my plans work.

In my world, food is medicine. My kitchen is my pharmacy, and my shopping list is my prescription pad. People come to me for help, to get them losing weight, when other methods have failed. They don't see how they will be camera-ready by Monday, or they need to blow through that last five pounds by Friday, or they absolutely have to look good in a bikini when the plane takes off for the beach at the end of the next week. They come to me when they have already lost ten, twenty, fifty, or seventy-five pounds, but their bodies have suddenly decided to rebel and stage a standoff. They come to me when they don't know what to try.

Sometimes they come to me with serious health issues. Doctors send people to me because they believe weight loss will help resolve infertility, diabetes, breast cancer, prostate cancer, depression and many other chronic health issues where weight gain is a catalyst. People come to me not just because they want to look good on the outside but because I can help them access the healing power of burning through food, toxins and fat. People put their trust in my methods, and if you are reading this book, thank you for putting your trust in them, too.

For those who aren't familiar with my programmes, I am a nutritional counsellor and registered wellness consultant with clinics in Beverly Hills and Burbank, California, as well as in Fort Collins, Colorado. I have more than twenty years of clinical experience using functional foods and natural therapies to effect targeted weight loss and heal the body from the inside out. I work with some of the world's leading physicians, fitness experts and chefs, as well as holistic health practitioners such as acupuncturists, reflexologists and herbalists. My clients are actors, musicians, professional athletes, medical patients, seniors, teenagers and parents. I couldn't possibly narrow down or put a label on my diverse and wonderful clients, but I can define what I do for them: my speciality is healing and sculpting bodies using food. I have advanced certifications in many different health disciplines, and I grew up in a holistic health environment. My mother is an acupuncturist, and my grandfather on my mother's side is Hopi, born and buried on the reservation. Using food as medicine and incorporating a variety of medicinal philosophies into everyday life has been in my family's blood for centuries, and I'm so excited that more people are finally grasping the medicinal power of food, herbs and teas.

I'm also a mom, with a blended family full of kids. We have busy lives just like yours. Monday is our most hectic morning, and that's the day we all have smoothies for breakfast. Each of my kids has his or her special recipe. (My daughter's smoothie always contains "lots of leaves".) On the other mornings, which move along at only slightly less than warp speed, I try to cook breakfast for everyone because I believe, from every minute of medical and health training I've ever had and with every ounce of my soul and spirit, that real food is the key to health, body management, energy and beauty. Food is the answer.

But the way I use food can vary drastically, depending on the problem at hand. I am a problem solver and a body detective. My speciality is how to apply food in strategic and exact ways in order to achieve highly specific results. In my clinic, people ask me how *The Burn* is different from *The Fast Metabolism Diet*. Whereas FMD is total rehab for your metabolism, *The Burn* is an intense and specific intervention into a blockage in your progress and health. For FMD, I selected foods for their micronutrient or glycaemic content, to rehabilitate your broken metabolism. It is a 28-day full-body metabolism overhaul, to be followed when your whole system needs repair. *The Burn* is completely different. It is another weapon in your arsenal against weight gain and poor health. Where the FMD is a blast of dynamite, *The Burn* is laser-focused on your weight loss plateaus and chronic health woes. Instead of choosing foods based on their micronutrients or glycaemic index, I've selected foods, herbs, teas, spices and food combinations on *The Burn* for their *thermogenic index,* or their ability to burn through the barriers that are keeping you from your goals. When something has stopped you in your tracks, *even if you think you have been doing everything right, The Burn* can intervene with a powerful microrepair for three specific system dysfunctions that can stall your weight loss:

1. Inflammation, which is a problem with your body's initial reaction to food.

2. Digestive dysfunction, which is a problem with your body's digestion of food.

3. Hormonal imbalance, which is a problem with your body's equilibrium between the production and biosynthesis of hormones.

This is a quick, intense, plateau-busting blaze that burns through your particular roadblock and scorches it in just three, five or ten days, depending on your barrier. No matter what has gotten in your way and hindered weight loss before, *The Burn* will help you burn right through it.

So if you're stuck, burn through it.

If you hit a plateau, burn through it.

If you want strategic weight loss, burn through it.

If you want to kick-start your weight loss plan, burn through it.

If you have water weight and inflammation, burn through it.

If you have gas and bloating, burn through it.

If you have hormone-based weight gain, for the love of God, burn through it!

THREE, FIVE OR TEN DAYS . . . REALLY?

Maybe you are a sceptic and you're wondering, "Can I really achieve total body transformation in three, five or even ten days?"

Indulge me. When you're through you're going to be dying to e-mail me your before-and-after pictures, but first let me explain why it is not only possible, but pretty darn easy to transform you in three short days, not to mention five or ten.

Let's pretend you're going out on a drinking binge. I'll go with you, to be your designated driver. First, we get all dressed up. It's Friday night and you're looking hot. You fix your hair, you put on a cute dress and heels (or a sharp suit), and you look at yourself in the mirror. Sexy!

Then you go out and start drinking. It's going to be the lost week-end. Maybe you kick it off with a good stiff martini. Then maybe you'll have some margaritas. In between rounds, have some bar food—you only live once! Nachos, loaded fries, buffalo wings, things like that. It'll be great—a blast. Order whatever you want! Throw caution to the wind. I'll get the next round.

You keep going, all through the night. Finally, afraid you'll pass out, I take you home. But as soon as you wake up, you're good to go again. Hair of the dog! Start with a mimosa. Then let's go have a three-martini lunch. It's Saturday night, so you're out on the town again. You might not look quite as sexy as you did on Friday night. A little bit mussed, a little bit swollen. Your hair is dry. Your skin sags a little. You have shadows under your eyes. But you are determined. Three days, remember? By Sunday night, you've slowed down considerably. Maybe you're just drinking beer now. Bottoms up! More fries? How about a burger? Or maybe all you can stomach at this point is a box of cookies and a wine cooler. By the time you go to bed on Sunday, you barely remember Friday.

Now, let's take a good look in the mirror first thing Monday morning. Do you think you would even resemble that person who was look-ing so hot on Friday night? Trust me, you don't. You're puffy. You're swollen. Those shadows under your eyes have turned into shiners, even if you didn't get into a single bar fight. Your belly bulges with bloat, your upper arms sag and, if you turn around, your cellulite is winking at you in the mirror. I think I see the beginning of a double chin. And can we talk about your breath?

But a drastic transformation doesn't have to be brought on by that extreme of an event. Have you ever had a Mexican-food-and-margarita morning? You know when you go out with friends and descend on the chip basket, order a big burrito and swill margaritas the whole night, you'll spend the whole next day sucking in your belly so your colleagues and friends don't think you've gone south of the border.

Have you ever had a ham hangover? You know those nights when you eat too much ham and wine, or bratwurst and beer, and you wake up bloated with sodium, you can't get your rings on, and your eyes are so puffy you hardly recognize yourself?

And if you're still at the bar when it's the "last call for alcohol", even if it's only one night, I can guarantee it will be stretchy pants and a big

T-shirt for you tomorrow because those skinny jeans you peeled off and threw on the floor last night won't fit after just one night of partying.

Have you ever woken up with "allergy shiners" or "adrenal shiners", those dark circles around your eyes and puffy bags under them? These are due to your adrenal glands reacting to something that either is an allergen for you or has become a stress reaction food. What I mean by that is that you have eaten a go-to food frequently when under stress. Mine happens to be ice cream. When you do this, your body becomes conditioned to release stress hormones because it associates that food with stress. Both of these situations can cause those dark circles—you don't have to be allergic to a food to have this reaction.

Have you ever had blurred vision or seen black spots in front of your eyes after an extreme sugar binge? In Chinese medicine, it is said that the liver *qi*, or energy, opens through the eyes. The liver is where the body stores excess sugar. They say that blurred vision is "the liver drowning in sweets".

What about post-holiday "Dunlap's disease"? Have you suffered from this one? This is when you throw all caution to the wind from Halloween to Super Bowl Sunday because there's no sense starting a diet until all the holiday parties and celebrations are over. Come February, you realize that your belly has dun lapped over your belt buckle.

But you don't need months to do a number on yourself, as you saw from our weekend jaunt. You don't even need days. All you really have to do to prove that the body can transform in just a few hours is to Google a picture of a celebrity all glammed up for an awards ceremony, looking taut and radiant and alive, and then Google their police mug shot eight to ten hours later. Take a good hard look at those before-and-after pics and just try to tell me that a little bit of time and effort can't dramatically change your appearance, not to mention rock your entire world.

Take everything you've just read and flip it on its head. Three days of bad behaviour can certainly make a dramatic difference. But let's look on the other side of the coin. Three days of highly targeted nourishing and body-activating *good behaviour* can make just as much of a difference. My friend the respected doctor and author Mark Hyman once wrote, "The fact is that most of us are only a few days away from having control over our bodies." This is exactly what I believe. If you can look *that bad* on Monday morning after a weekend of drinking and terrible food (or an overindulgent vacation or a bout of stress eating or a brutal round of PMS or menopausal symptoms), you can look *that good* on Monday morning after three days of targeted nutrition. Here's what we can do to you and your appearance, your energy level, your world: we can light it on fire.

Look, I'm all for going out and having a good time. Heck, I do it myself. But here's the thing. If you have the occasional glass of wine with friends on a Thursday evening, your body can handle that. But if you are missing work because of a hangover, you need an intervention. When your body has stopped being able to lose weight, it's just like that hangover. Something is wrong, and you've lost control. It's time to take it back. When your metabolism needs help, a little microrepair can change everything.

I will always explain the science behind what I'm doing. If you're as fascinated by that as I am, and if you love knowing exactly what you're getting into before you sign up, then you're going to love the first few chapters of this book. I will help you spot yourself and the problems you've been having with weight loss. We'll work together to determine which symptoms are troubling you the most and choose which issues you want to resolve first. After that, we'll jump right in—because your time is valuable and plateaus should be short-lived. You'll foil your weight loss plateau, no matter how much time you have to devote to burning your barriers down.

Ready, set, and go—you'll put your head down, dig in, plough through, and in three, five or ten days, you'll look up, look in the mirror, and you will experience that *wow* moment you've been waiting for. You're going to be smokin' hot, and you'll have everything you need to stay that way.

PART ONE

STRIKE THE MATCH

CHAPTER ONE

Why You Aren't Losing Weight

Sometimes—often, in fact—even in the best possible world, even with the best possible diet, weight loss stalls. The number on the scale stops before it gets to the place you want it to be. When you haven't lost the weight you need to lose, there is always a reason. Always. It is a scientific reason, and it has nothing to do with any personal failing on your part. It is not about willpower or weakness. It is about biochemistry. Stalled weight loss, especially under conditions where you are giving your body everything it needs to lose weight, is a sign that something has gone wrong in the system.

A tiny splinter in your big toe can cause a cascade of major problems throughout your entire body if you don't do something about it. But the solution isn't to cut off your foot. You have to pull out the splinter, but not carelessly, haphazardly, or in a way that does more harm than good. To pull out a splinter takes concentration, precision and the right tool.

When weight loss stalls, when you hit a plateau, your body is sending you a message. You have the equivalent of a splinter in your metabolic system. To get weight loss started again, you need to take tweezers to that splinter, carefully and skilfully, so your body can get back down to business doing what it does best: burning fat for fuel.

But how did you get that splinter? The way the body handles food is pretty amazing. If point A is eating and point Z is living, metabolism is all the letters in between. Metabolism is the rate at which we convert food into life. Like Rumpelstiltskin spinning straw into gold, metabolism spins food into you—into skin and hair and blood and bone and muscle and energy. It is the chemistry of life, and the magic that turns a meal on a plate into the life you live every moment of the day.

But this doesn't happen instantaneously. The transformation of food into life by the metabolism is a process. When you eat food, there are basically three things your body does with it:

1. Your body reacts to food.

2. Your body digests food.

3. Your body uses the micronutrients in food to create equilibrium between the production and biosynthesis of hormones.

At any point during this process—at the point of reaction to food, at the point of digestion of food, or at the point of hormone balancing—things can go wrong, and when that happens, the whole system breaks down. It's like that splinter in your toe—it seems like such a little problem, but if you don't deal with it, if you let it fester, then pretty soon, you might be in severe pain. You might not be able to walk or you might even get a systemwide infection. A small problem can quickly become a big problem, and in the case of the metabolism, a small problem at any point during the process can lead to swelling, bloating, acidity, inflammation, low energy, mood problems, weight gain, excessive fat accumulation, and even, eventually, chronic diseases such as arthritis, cancer, heart disease, autoimmune diseases and Alzheimer's. Metabolic problems are serious, and if you want to feel good and get rid of extra weight and fat, you need to deal with them.

The Burn is microrepair for the "splinter" in your metabolism. It focuses laserlike attention on the very specific source of your weight loss resistance so you can lose fat and weight rapidly. It is an intense intervention that can shatter your personal weight loss plateau. *The Burn* will incinerate the roadblocks that are holding you back from the body and health you desire. Use it strategically to reach your goal, whether that is to wow a crowd this weekend, zip your jeans by Friday, or resculpt your entire body into a more pleasing shape by next weekend. The core promise of *The Burn* is this: you can make a profound and dramatic change in your appearance, health and energy in just a few days.

And we will do it with food. Food is medicine, and it can help or harm the body, depending on how you use it.

WHAT *THE BURN* CAN DO FOR YOU

Maybe you are preparing for something, like a public appearance or a class reunion. Perhaps you are repairing *after* something, like holiday excess or a long weekend at an all-inclusive resort. Are you finishing your weight loss journey or just kicking it off? Maybe you are answering an SOS call from your skinny jeans or you have an eye on swimsuit season.

Maybe your doctor has even warned you that you need to lose weight or you are at risk of a health issue, such as prediabetes or infertility or fatty liver disease. My clients often come to me focused on the physical appearance they want and how their bodies will look once weight loss has been achieved, but the real miracle and power of weight loss is physically being in weight loss mode. Even if you lose just three or five pounds, when your body is in the process of losing weight, it makes drastic changes. You will have a shift in your inflammation, in the way you process micronutrients and in your hormones, as soon as you start the weight loss process. It's not just about looking amazing when you're done losing the weight (although that happens, too). It's about what you are promoting in your total health when you step out of the mode of weight gain or weight loss resistance and into weight loss.

This is what *The Burn* can do for you—launch you back into weight loss mode and back into the cascade of positive biochemical changes that affect your body. Whether you have a lot to lose or just a little, get ready for serious transformation.

One of the best things about *The Burn* is that it is something anyone can do. Whatever your food philosophy, dietary restrictions, habits or inclinations, *The Burn* can work for you. Step out of what you are doing for a few days and hand yourself over to me. Let me give you a jumpstart, and then you can drive on down the road, going back to what you were doing before. Maybe you live by *The Fast Metabolism Diet*. Excellent choice! Or maybe you are devoted to some other system—or no system at all. Maybe you fly by the seat of your pants. I hear that! There are many ways to live a healthy life.

That's another thing that makes this programme different—*The Burn* is not a way of life. It is not something to do forever. It is an intense and prescriptive tool to use for the purpose of metabolic micro-repair. Step in, shake things loose and then step back out again. It's your tool to use whenever you need it.

WHY AND HOW I USE FOOD AS MEDICINE

I didn't start out studying human nutrition. In fact, I didn't start out studying humans at all. I'm a die-hard aggie, which means I studied animal science. I believe that has always given me an edge. This area of study focuses intensively not just on nutrition but on how food can transform, in very specific ways, the ratio, distribution and composition of muscle and fat in a mammal's body.

I had a special knack for this in school. One of the assignments we used to have to do was to manipulate that muscle-to-fat ratio by adjusting an animal's feed. This fascinated me, and I quickly learned that how an animal eats can increase the kind of internal fat that results in heavy marbling, or can shrink the subcutaneous fat for a tighter, leaner, more defined look. I learned not just how to maximize weight gain in a short period of time, but how to maximize weight loss.

Animal science is a lot different from human medicine because you can't say to a sheep, "Do you feel better? Were you satisfied with the results of this medication? How are you feeling emotionally?" You can't get the same kind of feedback from an animal that you can from a human, so animal science and veterinary medicine have to measure results like no other industry. Another thing about aggies, or animal people, including farmers and horse people, is that they are supremely open-minded. We will try many different roads to get the results we want, and much of the work with animals today is preventive. We pull our strategies from all kinds of arenas and we try all kinds of therapies—acupuncture, massage, supplements, homeopathy, Chinese medicine, different ways of preparing foods from cooked to raw to processed—it's all about keeping the vet out of the barn! The goal is to have a stable full of animals that are at peak performance, able to reproduce easily, maintain an ideal body weight and have healthy coats and strong hooves.

If you see an animal with its ribs showing in the animal indus-try, we would consider that abuse. In the human world, however, we have the strange idea that this is beautiful. As a woman and a mom of daughters, I think this is sick. In the animal industry, it is obvious that nurturing, love, care, attention and good food beget a healthy animal. And we have no trouble treating our pets this way. But ourselves? No. Many will get up in the morning and feed their pets, and then walk out of the house without breakfast. All your dog or cat has to do is lie around and lick themselves, and you run out the door with huge ex-pectations for the day—and no breakfast. This is so crazy to me! In the human world, we consistently deprive ourselves and each other of what we need for glowing health, and then continue to abuse ourselves when we aren't healthy enough, beautiful enough, thin enough. Where is the disconnect? Why can't we treat ourselves the way we treat our beloved animals? We can, and *The Burn* is how you move in that direction.

When I decided not to become a veterinarian, it was partially due to curiosity. I came out of college knowing a whole lot about how to sculpt animal bodies, yet I couldn't help wondering whether what I learned in animal science would work on people. I didn't see why it wouldn't, so I began to study human nutrition, and I did so with a vastly open mind, like any good aggie. I've studied the Western system of health exten-sively, as well as with masters of many other systems. I have studied the Chinese philosophy of medicine, which looks at what foods affect certain organs, tissues, glands and systems. I consider the Ayurvedic perspective, which matches foods to certain body and energy types. I have studied the German philosophy of homotoxicology, which fo-cuses on how bodies toxify and detoxify. I've even studied the *Farmer's Almanac* because I've seen in my practice how the seasons affect the way our bodies process food. What time of year will you best benefit from raw foods, or cooked foods? When do you need more fat, and when do you need more vegetables? I ask myself questions like this all the time. I am on a never-ending quest for knowledge about how food affects the body.

For all these reasons, when I have a client with a weight loss issue, I am not likely to ask, "Is the problem insulin resistance?" or "Is this per-son just overeating?" Instead, I am more likely to ask, "Why is insulin resistance manifesting in this person's body?" or "Why is this person eating more than his body needs?" and "What systems can we nurture and repair to perfect the body's natural process, so the body can become functional again?"

My whole practice is based on this philosophy of open-mindedness, with the stringent expectation of results. I have relentlessly searched for the techniques that work, and wherever I find them, I pluck out the parts that make a difference in the human body, and I leave the parts that don't. I have no preconceptions about the validity of a health programme. I will try anything to heal, repair and transform the body. I'll scour the latest clinical trials published in medical journals and at the same time tie chicken bones around my neck and dance down the hallways of my clinic if it will get someone the results they need. I have only one requirement before I apply a technique, strategy or philosophy to my own practice: it has to work.

It *has to work*. I have clinics in some rough areas. My clients threaten me with knives—as in, "If this doesn't work, I'm going under the knife!" OK, this is mainly an issue in my Beverly Hills clinic, but the last thing I want is for someone to undergo plastic surgery when I know I can do "surgery" on them purely by manipulating their diet. The doctors who send their patients to me will stop sending them if I don't get their bodies and their numbers (cholesterol, blood sugar, hormone levels) under control. For many of my clients, weight loss is a matter of life and death. If I don't deliver, they don't heal. If I don't deliver, my celebrity clients will look elsewhere, too.

I expect major results from my clients' bodies. When those results stop happening, when they get stuck, I'm always looking at the *why*. When I figure out the *why*, then I go to my toolbox (consisting primarily of food), and I pull out what's going to get them unstuck. I pull out what will evoke real, clinical, tangible, visual results. It's always about the results.

People say I have a knack for knowing how to sculpt a body to exact specifications. They say I have secrets, and they're right. My secrets come from every corner of the globe and from every era in history. They become the secrets of my clients, and the longer you stay with me, the more of them you will learn. Soon you will know what I know, and it will transform you.

The teas and smoothies in the *Burn* plans are medicinal. Their job is to help you heal. Some people love 'em, and some people do not. If you fall into the "do not" category, don't worry. You can feel free to dilute either of them if they taste too strong, with water or with ice when using your blender. You can also add a natural flavouring or sweetener like stevia, xylitol, vanilla or cinnamon. Add directly to your tea or blend them into the smoothie. You could even add the tea or smoothie to your soup, if you like it better that way. Or just plug your nose and take your dose! We've got to get the job done, and the results will be worth it.

WHY THREE DIFFERENT *BURN* PLANS AND WHICH ONE IS RIGHT FOR YOU?

My clinic is like a research and development lab. I do R&D on people, and then I bring it to you. When I have the luxury of going one-on-one with someone, I can figure out exactly what they need and create a plan just for them. I do this all day, every day. And something that has always interested and challenged me the most was when clients who seemed to be doing fine suddenly stopped losing weight. My experience addressing these challenges provides the basis for the book you're holding in your hands and the information that will help you today.

I'm frequently called upon to provide results *immediately*. I love having the luxury of a full month, or at least two weeks, to get my clients to a good place. Often, I don't have that much time. Somebody has to start filming a movie in a week and a half, or appear on an awards show on Friday and it's already Monday, or has to look fantastic for a photo shoot on Monday, *when it's already Friday.*

I live for these situations—they bring out my inner Sherlock Holmes and my inner adrenaline junkie, too! I'm always up for the challenge, and when someone can't break through a plateau, I want to know why. Over the years, whenever this happened, I dug deeper, with questions and lab tests and a physical evaluation. The more I investigated, tested and learned, the more I saw the same patterns rearing their heads.

What I noticed was that weight loss plateaus are almost always caused by one of three different problems: inflammation, digestive issues or hormonal imbalance. Targeting these areas is not only the answer to the problem of the weight loss plateau, but *also* the key to high-speed body makeovers.

So when I get only three days with you, we target the body's *inflammatory* reactions to food, which cause swelling due to water and lymph retention. We focus on the kidneys, lymphatic system and bladder function. I flush out, detoxify and hydrate the body, producing prominent cheekbones, slim ankles and a radiant complexion. I call this the I-Burn.

When I get only five days with you, we target the body's backed-up *digestion* of food and clogged respiratory system by focusing on the mucosal lining of the digestive tract and lungs. This is how we look at it: the mucosal lining of the lung and large intestine are made from the same tissue. One allows oxygen to get into the bloodstream. The other allows micronutrients to get into the bloodstream. Oxygenation is crucial for the metabolism and to maintain blood pH and oxygen saturation in the blood. This is how the nutrients get broken down and taken to the mitochondria to fuel metabolism. I debloat the tummy, oxygenate the lungs and supercharge the circulation for a flat belly and tighter hips and thighs, and to give the body an abundance of energy. I call this the D-Burn.

When I get only ten days with you, we target the body's *hormone* system by focusing on using food to create balance. When hormones are out of balance, the body uses fat cells in two ways. One, to absorb hormones that are not properly broken down, and two, to produce hormones to try to create equilibrium. Both situations cause a proliferation of fat cells, or aggressive weight gain. I give you what you need to release and incinerate fat so you can manufacture and synthesize the hormones that will transform you from stuck to sexy. I call this the H-Burn.

Time and time again, I send my clients out the door with one of these three programmes, to break through their plateaus. Most of my clients have tried at least one, and often all three, of these methods multiple times throughout the years, and now you can try them, too. You're next! Let's transform you and turn you loose on the red carpets of the world. Maybe your red carpet, like mine, is on the sidelines of your child's football game. No matter where you are or what you are doing, it feels so good to put your best foot and best you forward. So what's the source of your weight loss resistance? In most cases, weight loss stalls for one of these three reasons:

- The body is holding on to excess fluid—water and lymph—in an attempt to mitigate reactivity by diluting toxicity. The slowdown in the body's natural systems of elimination causes a rise in acidity of the body's tissues and systemic inflammation. This in turn causes excess subcutaneous fat accumulation, or cellulite, as the body seeks to find places to store the toxins that are building up.

- The gastrointestinal system isn't working properly and is getting backed up. This also slows down another of the body's natural toxin elimination systems, causing the accumulation of thick, heavy, resistant yellow fat, as the body looks for additional toxin storage facilities.

- The micronutrients in the food you are eating aren't getting synthesized properly into the chemicals/hormones you need to keep your weight in check, causing aggressive accumulation of soft, fluffy, lumpy white fat, which takes on some of the characteristics of hormones and causes even further hormonal imbalance in your system.

Depending on which of these issues you are having, or which is causing you the most difficulty (many people have problems with more than one), you may choose whichever of the three *Burn* plans is most appropriate. Each will help you bust through a plateau, but direct you in a different way for achieving it. What you are doing hasn't been working. So instead of doing more of it (like exercising *more*) or less of it (like eating *less*), we are going to shake it up in order to turn things around.

Do you recognize yourself yet?

Maybe you already have an idea that you aren't reacting to foods correctly. If that's you, you need to become an I-Burner in the battle against fluid accumulation, subcutaneous fat and inflammation.

If you relate to having digestive issues, respiratory issues, or thickening of your body, or if you've developed hard rolls of fat in easy-to-find places, then you need to dig deep, becoming a D-Burner who can burn through those digestive blockages and excavate that heavy, thick fat accumulating all over your body.

If you understand exactly what I mean about hormone-based weight gain—if you are aggressively gaining weight and your shape is changing in a way you don't like, and you are having roller-coaster emotions—then you need to become an H-Burner so you can stop the aggressive weight gain, guide your hormones back into balance, and start burning off that excess fat to sculpt your shape into the form it's meant to take.

No matter which you choose, you will be doing something great for your body:

- When you do the I-Burn, you will fight your body's reactivity to food. In three days, you could lose up to three pounds. After you conquer your foes and win your battle, you will be likely to hear comments like, "Wow, your skin looks fantastic!" or "You look so pretty today!" or "You look so well rested and healthy." Three pounds carved from the right areas of your body can make a drastic change in your appearance.

- When you do the D-Burn, you will unearth the issues with your body's digestion of food. In five days, you could lose up to five pounds. Once you've struck gold, you're likely to hear comments like, "Gosh, your waist is tiny!" and "Your stomach is so flat!" and "You look so healthy!" Imagine a five-pound blanket covering your entire body. Now imagine unwrapping it and throwing it off. That's the difference you can make in five days.

- When you do the H-Burn, you will create harmony in your hormones to resculpt your body. In ten days, you could lose up to ten pounds. You'll evoke comments like, "OMG, how much weight have you lost?" and "Your body shape has *completely changed.*"

There are many good reasons to choose any particular plan. All of them will benefit you, so it's not like you can possibly choose the wrong one, but consider which one appeals to you most. Here are some additional things to consider:

1. WHAT ARE YOUR PHYSICAL ISSUES?

Maybe you are flexible in your schedule and you want to base your decision on what the plan will do for you. You can certainly choose based on your own particular weight loss barrier. The next three chapters will get into depth about what each plan addresses, but here is a summary to get you thinking in the right direction:

- Swelling, puffiness and bumpy cellulite accumulation suggest you should do the I-Burn for three days, to nurture the kidneys, lymphatic system and bladder; liquefy and flush subcutaneous fat; cool inflammation and release water weight.

- Hard yellow fat accumulation in the belly and around the rib cage, stomach bloating, digestive issues, and respiratory issues such as a cold or a cough suggest you should do the D-Burn for five days, to repair and relax the mucosal lining, ease digestion and burn away that yellow fat.

- Hormonal imbalance, moodiness, and aggressive fat accumulation in strange places that make your body look disproportionate—a muffin top, chubby knees, upper back fat—suggest you should do the H-Burn, to nourish and stabilize the liver, gallbladder and thyroid in order to repair and balance the system that manufactures and regulates hormone production. We are taking that job away from the pesky and intrusive fat cells by disintegrating and releasing them. Remember, when our hormonal equilibrium is off, we create fat stores to absorb excess hormones and then create additional fat cells to produce accessory hormones, creating a dysfunction in equilibrium.

And if you checked "all of the above" and every symptom I talk about here and in the next three chapters sounds like you? Then just pick any of the plans. They are all supremely nourishing and therapeutic. Or address your worst problem first, and then you can see where you are and decide what you might want to do next.

Many of my clients come to me with multiple issues. We choose a plan based on which issues are the most troubling at the time. If you aren't even sure what problem you want to address, just pick one. The plan will nourish and support you. When you're done, you will have addressed one area and then you can reassess to determine what issues to tackle next. You can't choose the wrong plan.

2. HOW MUCH TIME DO YOU HAVE?

I wish that your answer were "As much time as I need to repair what's gone awry in my body." But I know how it goes. I get those calls three days before the Academy Awards: "Help me! I have to look fabulous in my Valentino gown on Sunday!" If you've only got a weekend, then the decision is easy: you will be my I-Burner, flushing out excess fluid and subcutaneous fat for super-quick results. But if you have to look good by *next* weekend, then maybe you are a D-Burner. You can take a few more days to dig a little deeper and tackle any roadblocks in your digestion, debloating your tummy and tightening up your curves. And if you've got more time to spare for total body transformation? Thank you! You are my dream client. You have time to do any of the three plans according to what your symptoms are, including the powerful H-Burn plan, to put your hormones back into balance and turn fat accumulation into fat burning.

I must make clear one caveat: if you choose a plan based on symptoms, then you must do the plan for the specified number of days, rather than choosing the number of days and then picking a plan to match your schedule. For example, if you solely identify with the H-Burn, you're going to have to give me those ten days. Don't try to sneak the H-Burn or even a D-Burn into a three-day slot. Three days is not long enough to get your digestion or your hormones unstuck, but it's the perfect amount of time to tackle inflammation.

The reason you can be successful choosing a plan based solely on your time frame is twofold. First, many people have at least some issue with each of these systems, and if you have some inflammation and some digestive issues and some hormonal issues, any of the plans will help you make progress and shake yourself loose from a plateau. Second, your body is a blend of all of these systems working together to form a whole, and that whole is you! Supporting any one of them with any of these nourishing, health-supporting plans will support the entire system and, in turn, every individual part of it.

If you're really stuck, though, focusing intensely on the one system that is giving you the most trouble, and doing so for the amount of time it takes, is the most precise and intensive way to get unstuck. I use this example with my clients: let's say you're in pain. An anti-inflammatory can help relieve your pain by addressing your entire system. But if your leg is broken, you'd better get yourself to an orthopaedic surgeon to get it repaired.

Doing a plan according to your schedule, even if the issue that plan addresses isn't a particular problem for you, is like taking that anti-inflammatory. Because all your systems work together as a whole, a whole-system-nourishing plan will make you feel better than you did before. Yet if you want to get down to the precise and exact reason why you are having weight loss resistance, then that is like treating the broken leg. You need a specialist, and you need the plan that will address your particular issue, no matter how long it takes. Would you tell your doctor that you only have three days to heal your broken leg?

So choosing a *Burn* plan according to your own schedule is like taking an anti-inflammatory. Choosing a *Burn* plan according to your physical issues is like visiting the surgeon. The intensity of your results is up to you and the time you are willing to make for yourself.

3. HOW MUCH WEIGHT DO YOU NEED TO LOSE?

Another way to choose a plan is to base your decision on how much you need to lose. Are you a little bit stuck? A lot stuck? Or is your current weight apparently cemented in stone? If you only want to lose three pounds, or quickly move past a new plateau, do the I-Burn. If you want to get rid of those last five pounds for good or bust through a more stubborn plateau, then do the D-Burn. If you need to lose ten pounds or more, or obliterate a plateau you've been fighting against for years, then go all the way and do the H-Burn. The reason behind this approach: the symptoms I see with my clients. Usually, if you are only three pounds away from your weight loss goal, it's an issue of inflammation or reaction. If you have a digestive issue, you almost always have more than three pounds to lose, and if you are manifesting hormone imbalance, your weight gain is typically ten pounds or more. If you have much more than ten pounds to lose, I suggest you begin with the H-Burn, because even if you have inflammatory and digestive issues, getting your hormones into balance first will repair your biggest issue.

4. WHAT DO YOU HAVE ON HAND?

When you go through the next few chapters and read the descriptions of all three plans in detail and you feel like your body is saying, "That's me, that's me, that's me," to all three plans and you know you are going to participate in all three plans at some point, another way to choose where to start is to look at the grocery lists and see what you have on hand. Do you have a garden full of courgettes or cucumbers or a lemon tree or grapefruit tree that's about to fall over? You will see, when you get to the plans, that you will need a ton of lemons and courgettes in the I-Burn plan, for example, or grapefruit galore in the H-Burn plan. Choose according to your food surpluses and you will save money while also getting great results in your body.

So what do you think? Which plan speaks to you? Each has its specific mechanisms for weight loss, metabolism repair and healing in various parts of the body, and Chapters 2, 3, and 4 will go into more detail about how each *Burn* plan accomplishes this. Read each of these chapters carefully, then make your choice. Again, don't worry about making the wrong choice—you can always do another plan at another time. They are all here for you, now and for the rest of your life.

Once you've determined where you want to start to best incinerate *your* trouble spots and get your metabolism and your weight loss moving again, I'll walk you through your plan step by step, meal by meal, and day by day. We'll buy and prep everything you need before you start. After that, it will be easy. All you have to do is follow your I-Burn, D-Burn or H-Burn plan, and you'll be burning it up.

Once you have chosen a plan, make space for it in your life and consider it sacred. You get to be active, not passive. Get excited about what's coming. Get inspired. This is a *big event* in your life, but unlike some events you might plan, this one won't result in five extra pounds or a hangover. You're going to feel great, so this is worth some major anticipation and dedication. Fight for those days, change some plans, and don't just go along with what everybody else wants you to do if it doesn't fit in with what you are doing for yourself right now. For the next three, five or ten days, you are getting yourself back. *The Burn* won't take a long time, but its work is profound and it deserves all your attention. Your world now works around it. No negotiation.

The food is incredible. The recipes are easy. The smoothies are succulent. The teas are rejuvenating. The soups are comforting. None of it will be unpleasant. I'm not interested in forcing you to suffer just to be skinny. I'm not an advocate of the "who cares what happens to your body as long as you are thin" school of thought. Instead, we are all about repair. I want to know what's wrong, and then I want to fix it, so your body can find its way back to its healthiest weight and most beautiful form without coercion, force and damaging practices.

But I do want you to be aggressive about the repair. Support your body in this life you're given, so you can live with vibrancy, energy and passion. If you're stuck, burn through it, fast and furious. That's what I can do for you, and what you can do for yourself. Once you learn how, you can always return to any of these plans when you need them.

This book is a way of extending my clinic and client experience to you, the reader who may not be able to come to my office to book an appointment. If you are ready to burn through your weight loss resistance, blast fat fast, douse your inflammation, obliterate your bloat and trim your silhouette, then hand yourself over to me. You're going to feel *The Burn*, and you're going to come out on the other side smouldering.

I have clients who have been with me for over twenty years. Do you know how many tricks those people have? Everything you learn for whatever plan you do can be used as you see fit after you finish it. My clients know just about everything I know, and now you are one of them. I want you to start developing a repertoire so you always know how to handle every situation. Retaining water? Pick up the I-Burn tools again. Feeling bloated? Revisit the D-Burn. Hormonal? Don't forget that the H-Burn is always available to you. Keeping *The Burn* in your life for whenever you need it will inspire and fire your metabolism so it stays alive and thriving and burning food for fuel.

If you haven't read *The Fast Metabolism Diet* yet, it's waiting for you. If you don't have *The Fast Metabolism Diet Cookbook* yet, you have many delicious treats in store. If you haven't visited my website yet, I welcome you. But right now, you and I have work to do. It won't take long, but when we're in it together, we need to be *in it*. Your body is an incredible machine, and under good conditions it works pretty darn well. But right now you've got a splinter, and we're going in with the surgical tools to remove it as smoothly and effortlessly as possible. Something is limiting your rate of burn—but not for long. The body you want is as simple as the foods you choose. What do you need to become your leanest, healthiest, sexiest you? Let's find out and let's unleash *your* burn.

CHAPTER TWO

Is Inflammation Causing Your Weight Loss Resistance?

Welcome to my office. Are you in need of the I-Burn?

If you were my client, and you came to my office for help losing weight, I would spend the first forty-five minutes of our visit talking about your symptoms. I would ask you how you are feeling, and what's bothering you, so I could help you decide what course of action you need to take to solve your problems. When you walk in, I don't have a preconceived idea of which plan is right for you. This is our time to decide what's wrong, and how you're going to turn this ship around.

This is just what happened with a client I'll call Jim. Jim came into my clinic to lose weight. He wanted to go on one of my cleanse programmes (these are highly structured and individualized plans that incorporate food and my products, such as shakes and supplements, for intensive weight loss). Jim is a movie producer and I've worked with him before. He'd had great success in the past, but he admitted that he'd been eating a lot of candy over the holidays, and he hadn't worked out once. "I pretty much haven't moved, except to reach for more food," he said.

Although he claimed to be ready for the cleanse, I took one look at the inflammation in his face and his swollen hands and said, "I've got an idea. Before we do it, let's do the I-Burn." I gave him the recipes for his I-Burn Smoothie, I-Burn Tea, and I-Burn Soup. "Make these up ahead of time and have them according to this schedule," I said. "Just follow the plan." He took one look at the list of foods and said, "I can do this! This looks great!"

Three days later, Jim was a changed man. He already looked like he'd done the whole cleanse. His system had been gummed up by his bad behaviour, but following the I-Burn cleared things out and got him primed for even more success.

So let's talk about you. Let's talk about what's going on with your body. I often get clients telling me things like, "Well, my ankles are swollen, but I'm sure that has nothing to do with my weight gain," or "I feel so puffy in the morning, but that's probably irrelevant." To me, nothing is irrelevant. I want you to be thinking about all of it. You're the one who walks around with your body all day every day. You're the one who's with you 24/7. All day long, your body is talking to you, and it's giving you subtle clues and hints to your imbalances. A lot of my clients come into my office believing that weight loss is about calories and portion sizes and that's about it, but to me, everything is a clue about why you are stuck. Everything you tell me means something to me.

SIGNS YOU NEED THE I-BURN

So let's look at your symptoms in detail. Think about everything that your body tells you that you don't like, and check all of the following that apply to you now or recently:

- ❏ Is your face puffy? Are your cheekbones Missing in Action?
- ❏ Do your arms and legs feel thicker than they should?
- ❏ Are your socks leaving marks around your ankles?
- ❏ Do you have puffy bags and/or dark circles under your eyes?
- ❏ Are you having trouble getting your rings off at the end of the day?
- ❏ Are your muscles hidden under swelling, oedema and cellulite?
- ❏ Have you noticed fat accumulating around your lower back, hanging over your pants?
- ❏ Are your underarms feeling chubby, sticking out from your short sleeves in lumps?
- ❏ Are your knees getting dimpled?

- ❑ Are your extremities tingling?
- ❑ Do you look pale?
- ❑ Are you feeling dehydrated, even though you keep drinking water?

If you checked more than half of these, then get the I-Burn onto your schedule. If you checked almost all of them, then what are you waiting for?

This plan will benefit you in many ways. It will make a rapid change in your face because everything you do is designed to torch fat and take the swelling down, and swelling tends to happen first in the face. This is one reason why this three-day plan will make you look and feel so much better. You could go from haggard-looking to picture-perfect in just a few days.

If you only need to lose a few pounds, or you just want to get the "fluff" off your body, this is another reason to do the I-Burn. If you need to show your upper arms and you don't want them puffy and wobbling, you can tighten them with the I-Burn. If you want to look younger and more radiant, do the I-Burn. If you've been retaining water lately—if you notice that you can gain two or three pounds overnight after a salt-heavy meal—then you need the I-Burn.

OTHER SIGNS YOU NEED THE I-BURN: YOUR MOOD

There are other, more subtle signs that the I-Burn plan is for you. In Chinese medicine, the kidneys are related to spontaneity and impulsivity. These can both be positive or negative qualities, depending on how you use them and how much control you have over them. You might be spontaneous and decide to take off on a vacation at a moment's notice. You might suddenly decide to buy that expensive handbag, or make a radical career change, or cut off all your hair. If you are in harmony, then there will be creativity in your spontaneity. It can make your life charming and fun. But if you are in disharmony, your impulsivity can become detrimental and cause dysfunction in your life.

I look at this aspect when evaluating my clients, but you can evaluate yourself. If you notice you are in a constant state of reactivity—you are making rash decisions you regret, or you are quick to fly off the handle or burst into tears or bite someone's head off, then you might have stressed kidneys. You may be blaming this on hormonal issues, but it could be reactivity. If you are feeling reactive, frenetic, tapped out, and like you don't have total control over what you are going to say and do next, then consider the I-Burn. I like to tell my clients, "If you are making rash decisions, or if you have a rash on your body, you need to do an I-Burn." This is the way to attack reactivity on all levels: emotionally and physically.

IS INFLAMMATION CAUSING YOUR WEIGHT LOSS RESISTANCE?

Now let's look a little more closely at what's really going on in your body if inflammation is the cause of your weight loss resistance. It all begins with reactivity.

As soon as you smell food, see food, or taste food, your body reacts. Even before you get down to the business of digestion, the first level of that reaction is immediate. This is why a child who is extremely allergic to peanuts can get a serious reaction just touching or even smelling peanuts. If you are allergic to a food or have an intolerance—if your body doesn't like it for any reason—then your face or throat might swell, your skin might break out in a rash or your stomach might rebel. It's like your body is declaring war on your food.

But reactions to food can be much less dramatic than this. Eat a food and if you are intolerant to it or already sensitive because you have a high load of toxicity, your lymphatic system and kidneys have to filter out all the parts that your body doesn't like. Or, eat a food full of agricultural chemicals or additives or fake processed ingredients, and your body has to do something with all the junk it can't use. The kidneys and lymphatic system are the central processing stations for enemy neutralization, and they are the first major organs to be impacted by what you eat. If your body sees that food as an enemy, in a dramatic or in just a subtle way, then it has to rescue you from that enemy.

Your kidneys filter every drop of your blood about every fifty minutes. According to the National Kidney Foundation, at the end of a twenty-four-hour period, your hardworking kidneys have filtered over two hundred litres of blood. That means food affects the kidneys, as well as the lymphatic system, very quickly—and we can impact these systems quickly too, just by changing what you are eating. A single meal with the right combinations of micronutrients or the wrong foods that cause reactivity in your system can affect your kidney function in less than an hour—for better or for worse.

The kidneys regulate water retention in your body and, as you now know, filter out toxins in the foods you eat. If your food is clean and pure and nourishing to the kidneys, all is well. The kidneys will do their job efficiently, with minimal stress, purging water and unused elements into the bladder and out when you pee. It's a beautiful system.

However, if your food is highly processed or contains toxic elements such as agricultural chemicals or if you drink alcohol, then your kidneys have to work a lot harder. In fact, I would even say they have to battle. Over time, a poor diet and other toxic exposure, along with other detoxification-slowing influences such as chronic stress, can increase the acidity of the body and overwhelm the kidneys (especially if they aren't receiving reinforcements in the form of good-quality fuel from the micronutrients in whole food). Under such conditions, the kidneys slow down; they aren't as effective. As kidney processing efficiency decreases, all those toxins that would normally get shuttled through in a timely manner start to build up and increase in concentration, threatening your defences.

Under these conditions, three things happen in your body:

1. Your lymphatic system, which is your body's drainage system, stops draining and holds on to water, in order to dilute the concentration of toxins in your body that are causing so much trouble. The more diluted they are, the less harm they can do, but all this water retention makes you swell up like a balloon.

2. In response to increased toxicity and acidity, your body triggers systemwide inflammation. Inflammation is normally a protective mechanism. It stimulates healing, as when you get an injury. However, too many toxins in your system, acidity (low pH in your tissues) and stress can all cause chronic long-term inflammation, which is destructive. When your body senses an overload of toxic material, an accumulation of fluid, and inflammation in

the system, it is programmed to send out a distress call that says, *stop burning fat*. Because toxins are typically stored in fat cells, burning fat releases even more toxins into the system. This happens all the time, and normally your kidneys can handle it. But if the system is already overloaded—if you are already at war, internally—then your body doesn't want to make the situation worse by burning any more fat.

3. Now that your body contains higher levels of waste than it should, it reacts by quickly shuttling that waste where it will do the least harm: straight into your fat cells. At the same time, your body sends another message: *make more fat cells*. These are the storage facilities for the toxins the kidneys haven't gotten around to processing and eliminating yet, and the more toxins you have, the more fat cells you need.

So at this point, you will be showing signs of fluid accumulation. You are holding on to water—your face looks puffier, your cheekbones disappear, your ankles swell, your socks leave marks on your legs, your hands look bigger and your rings get harder to put on and take off. You can also accumulate fluid around the lymph nodes—your knees get puffy, your underarms look fat and you can even get swollen jowls, so your face loses definition.

You will also begin to store subcutaneous fat in specific places. You can get fat pads under your eyes, fat pads on the backs of your knees, and fat pads around your lower back—that fat that hangs over the back of your jeans. You can even get dimples of cellulite on your stomach. "Kidney fat", as I call it, since kidney dysfunction is at the root of this particular type of fat accumulation, is squishy and dimply because it is right under the skin.

Basically, what is happening here is that your body is looking for little spots to store fat, so it can tuck away those toxins where they can't harm your vital organs, until the kidneys can get back on track again. If you don't do something to reverse this process, the cellulite will just keep piling on, and your body will become increasingly resistant to getting rid of it.

The effects of inflammation will be evident, too. Your skin will look ruddy and coarse. You might develop dark circles under your eyes, exaggerated by those new fat pads. You will look tired, even haggard, and definitely older.

So what are you going to do about it?

THE I-BURN: INFLAMMATION INTERVENTION

If you are reading all this and crying, "Yes, yes, yes!" then you need an intervention, and the one best suited to your situation is the I-Burn. This is three days of total body transformation. You will take down swelling in your face, limbs, armpits, knees and back related to excess toxin storage in your tissues. You will flush out the fluid your body has been collecting, and you will get rid of the subcutaneous fat known as cellulite. In just three days, you're going to look tighter, slimmer and younger. And plateaus? A distant memory.

WHAT YOU WILL ACHIEVE ON THE I-BURN

Now let's look at what's going to happen when you do the I-Burn, to motivate you to jump in and do what you need to turn yourself around. The I-Burn targets your body's reaction to food by nourishing and restoring the organs and systems that manage toxin removal: your kidneys, lymphatic system and bladder. Remember, your kidneys filter all the blood in your body in just under an hour—this means we can get a lot done in three days. This is a high-speed toxin purge that is designed to reduce oedema and scavenge cellulite, and the result will be fast, effective weight loss. You can lose up to three pounds in three days. You will also:

- Create an excretion reaction, which means your body starts flushing rather than holding on to toxins. If left circulating, these toxins will increase acidity in the body and signal the body to halt fat metabolism and create more fat cells for toxin storage.

- Hydrate your body to dilute toxins, and help the kidneys work more easily to flush them out instead of creating fat cells to store them.

- Deluge the body with kidney-supportive micronutrients from bitter foods such as beetroot tops and watercress, and white foods such as Asian pears and cabbages, as well as targeted thermogenic herbs, spices, teas and smoothies.

- Make the body more alkaline. A stable pH increases the rate at which the body metabolizes, or burns through, food. On the I-Burn, the intense levels of active enzymes and phytonutrients in the large portions of raw fruits and vegetables will positively impact the pH of your body.

- Provide low amounts of easy-to-digest protein sources through-out the day, largely consisting of nuts, seeds and legumes (prefer-ably raw and sprouted) as well as small amounts of cooked animal proteins, limited to turkey, eggs and fish (preferably raw). How-ever, note that you never *have to* eat animal protein on this plan. You can be completely vegetarian or vegan on the I-Burn.

With the I-Burn, you will attack subcutaneous fat (cellulite and oedema), stabilize your body's pH and reduce inflammation. We'll quickly smooth out the lumpy bumpies, deflate the swelling, soothe the bags under your eyes, return your hands and feet to their normal size, and ignite your glow. There is no way you're going to stay stuck once you've achieved these significant changes in your body.

WHY YOU WILL LOSE WEIGHT ON THE I-BURN

Three days doesn't sound like a lot for significant weight loss. Oh, but it is! Because the kidneys' reaction to food is so rapid, three days is a long time to nourish and support that system. As you target the lymphatic system with the foods and practices on this plan, you will get fluid moving again, so it can dump the fat cells into the bloodstream for the kidney to filter and the bladder to excrete. Bye-bye cellulite!

You are going to lose weight because we are going to turn off the signals that tell the body to stop weight loss: inflammation and acidity. When you bring down acidity and stabilize pH, and dilute toxins with deep hydration, you will turn off inflammation, increase the blood flow to the subcutaneous fat, and activate the lymphatic system to pump toxins out of the fat and into the bloodstream, where the kidneys can filter them and the bladder can excrete them. This tells your body that it's OK to kick-start fat burning again, and that equals serious weight loss.

Those sock rings around your ankles, those stuck rings around your fingers, that puffy face, those eye bags, are not random symptoms. They are telling you something. They are distress calls from your body. I'm not the only one telling you that your pH is off, that toxins are building up, that your kidneys aren't efficient and that you have inflammation—these are all talking to you. Your rings, socks and face are telling you that you need help detoxifying. If you are in a state of inflammation and reaction, your body is telling you that you have not had enough detoxification support. Your body is calling for the I-Burn, and you need to step up and send those bags under your eyes packing.

YOUR I-BURN PLAN: WHAT TO EXPECT

Now you might be thinking: "I hear you, socks. I hear you, rings. I hear you, eye bags. But how do I burn through the problem?" I'm here to tell you.

Here is your mission: you need to reduce your body's reactivity so you can excrete toxins more efficiently. This will show your body that it no longer needs to store fat, and that it can start burning it again. You're going to increase your rate of burn, and these are your tools. Every one of them supports, nourishes and facilitates the function of the kidneys, lymphatic system and/or bladder. They are all required parts of your I-Burn battle plan. What we are doing here is complex, and failing to bring any of these tools to the job can leave a vital area unsupported and become a rate-limiting factor in weight loss. For the most complete and dramatic win, do not skip anything.

You'll get to eat five times every day so you won't be hungry, and you'll be giving your body everything it needs to shed everything you don't want.

Let's take a closer look at each of the I-Burn components.

I-Burn Smoothie: You'll start every day with this delicious smoothie full of blueberries and cranberries, cucumber and lime, walnuts and rich avocado. You won't believe how good it tastes, or how well it kicks off your day. The purpose of the I-Burn Smoothie is to stabilize your pH, bringing down acidity and thereby reducing inflammation, so your body stops sending the signal to hold on to fat, fluid and weight.

I-Burn Tea: You will drink this tea throughout the day, savouring the citrusy lemon taste with its subtly savoury undertones of parsley and celery seed and its kick of cayenne pepper to get your metabolism moving. Its primary purpose is to dilute toxins, which will reduce their inflammatory effects, and promote rapid and efficient excretion of those toxins, to get them out of your body.

I-Burn Soup: You will eat this soup at least twice per day. Full of filling root veggies, sweet potatoes, mushrooms and greens, this soup intensely nurtures the kidneys, lymphatic system and bladder by delivering micronutrients that support them.

I-Burn Recipes: Use the I-Burn recipes for lunches and dinners in the recipe chapter, to add to your soup and tea for each of these meals. These are strategically designed with particular thermogenic combinations of herbs and spices to increase the blood flow to subcutaneous fat. This intense vasodilation is like reaching in and grabbing that fat and excess fluid from your tissues, so you can excrete it, but you'll do it painlessly with yummy meals such as Hummus Coleslaw, Roasted Vegetables on Courgette "Pasta" and Mexican Dinner Salad.

Water: On the I-Burn, you will drink half your body weight in ounces of water every day. This is a crucial weapon because dilution is the solution to pollution. Deep hydration lightens the burden on the kidneys by diluting the toxins.

I-Burn Success Boosters: Success Boosters are supportive therapies I use in my clinics that I have pulled from many different systems over my years of study. They include exercise options as well as herbs, teas, therapies, easy boosts and more intense boosts.

GET YOUR CALENDAR

If this is the plan for you, go and get your calendar right now, whether it's the family wall calendar, your appointment book or your smartphone. Whatever you use to keep track of the must-dos on your schedule, grab it and let's take a look.

It is very important that you make a time commitment to take three days and do everything on the plan. Clear the space. Cancel plans that you know will interfere. Carve out the time and commit. I am serious. Would you schedule a lunch meeting on the day of your wedding, or a night out with your friends when your big presentation at work is first thing in the morning? No, you have priorities, and *The Burn* is your priority now.

Even if you think the I-Burn is for you, read the next two chapters about the conditions and situations that make the D-Burn or H-Burn most appropriate. I want you to start in the place that is best for you right now. If you are really sure you want to begin with the I-Burn, go straight to Chapter 5 and jump right in.

CHAPTER THREE

Is Digestion Causing Your Weight Loss Resistance?

If you were to come into my office wondering about the D-Burn, or if the first thing you mentioned to me about yourself was any sort of digestive distress, I would sit you down and we would talk about your symptoms, just as we did when evaluating the I-Burn. This time, I would be looking for some different kinds of manifestations that you are having in your weight loss resistance. Because the D-Burn is all about the mucosal lining, in terms of both digestion and respiration, I would have an ear out for any symptoms related to those systems, as all of it could potentially be relevant to our analysis of whether you need the D-Burn.

But sometimes, digestive and/or respiratory issues aren't the first problem that comes up. Often, the issue is the plateau. That's what happened with my client Jean. When I first met Jean, she weighed 208 pounds, which was too much for her five-foot, five-inch frame. She told me she had lost weight and gotten down to 165 pounds several times in her life, but that was where she always hit a plateau. I evaluated her situation and put her on the FMD (*Fast Metabolism Diet*) because after years of chronic dieting, her metabolism needed major repair. Lo and behold, she got down to 165, but then, for no apparent reason, she stopped losing weight. That plateau had reared its ugly head again. She kept bouncing around between 167.5 and 164.9 but couldn't break through. She felt incredible, her hair looked great, she had tons of energy and she was just in love with this way of eating, but she couldn't figure out why she had stopped shy of the weight she always thought should be hers: 145.

Then she mentioned something that gave me an idea. She was having some digestive issues, such as bloating after eating. Perhaps that plateau was caused by a glitch in her digestion. I recognized that Jean needed *The Burn* to break through this stubborn plateau, so we decided she should do the D-Burn.

After five days, Jean reported that the bloating had disappeared, and she began to lose weight again. She had re-entered weight loss mode, and so I put her back on FMD. She began to lose weight rapidly after that. Just last week, Jean called to tell me that the scale had finally hit her magic number. She now weighs 145 pounds and she's exactly where she always knew she should be.

SIGNS YOU NEED THE D-BURN

Now it's your turn. Let's look more closely at the symptoms you've been having lately. Think about what your body is telling you. What are the subtle (or not-so-subtle) messages? Are any of them on the following list? Check all those that apply to you now or recently.

- ❑ Is your belly bloated? Do you notice bloating after eating meals?
- ❑ Are you having more gas than usual, or in an amount that seems excessive to you? (Everyone has gas, but it shouldn't be bothering you all day long.)
- ❑ Are you constipated, or having bouts of diarrhoea, or alternating between constipation and diarrhoea?
- ❑ Have you been diagnosed with IBS (irritable bowel syndrome) or do you have what you think of as a "nervous stomach"?
- ❑ Do you have heartburn or indigestion once a week or more often?
- ❑ Does your toilet bowl look like a salad bowl, with visible undigested food in your stool?
- ❑ Do your fat stores feel hard and dense? Is your stomach

protruding, or do you have thick, hard rolls around your waistline?

❑ Do you feel like you have a thick, heavy blanket of fat all over your body that isn't supposed to be there—like the "real you" is definitely smaller all over than you appear right now?

❑ Do you have mental fog and fatigue?

❑ Do you have tiny white bumps on the backs of your arms?

❑ Is your skin breaking out, or does it look crinkly and old?

❑ Do you have mucus in the back of your throat, or are you coughing up phlegm? Do you have a feeling of chronic congestion in your sinuses or lungs?

❑ Does your tongue have a thick white coat on it?

If you checked about half of these, then you need to make an appointment with your digestive tract. If you checked almost all of them, your mucosal lining is definitely trying to get your attention.

If you want to feel really good in your own skin, move more easily and reclaim your flat stomach, then it's time for the D-Burn. If you want to break through a plateau and that extra all-over layer of fat that makes you feel bigger than you really are, it's time for the D-Burn. If you need to clear your mind and your lungs and your colon, then it's definitely time for the D-Burn. If you sit down to dinner with a flat stomach and leave the table looking three months pregnant, then the D-Burn is the plan for you.

OTHER SIGNS YOU NEED THE D-BURN: YOUR MOOD

There are many physical signs that spell "D-Burn, please!" but other symptoms are more subtle but just as urgent. In many philosophies of medicine, particularly Eastern philosophies like Chinese medicine and Ayurveda, what happens in your body can be reflected in your emotions. I find that people who need the D-Burn often have particular types of mood signs. If you feel stuck or stagnant, or if your mind feels thick and slow, like you have mental phlegm, it means the digestive and respiratory systems in the body need some attention. The D-Burn is just the plan for this. If you find yourself taking a hard, harsh, stubborn stance on things that normally wouldn't matter all that much to you, then this is also a sign that you need the D-Burn. When you don't feel the breath of life in you because you feel foggy, fat and fatigued; if you've had to loosen your bra straps lately; if your pants are cutting off your circulation; if you feel like you've turned from a ballerina into a linebacker, or if you just feel stagnant and stuck, then you definitely need the D-Burn.

IS DIGESTION CAUSING YOUR WEIGHT LOSS RESISTANCE?

If the D-Burn sounds like it might be the plan for you, I want you to understand what's really going on in your body right now. It all begins with the mucosal lining.

When you eat food, it goes on a journey, deep down through your body. Your first exposure to a food can cause inflammation, and when this happens, I usually suspect that the I-Burn is in order because it is a fast-acting plan. After your initial reaction to food, as you begin to digest it and your body begins to assimilate the nutrients, you can experience some other problems. These are primarily related to the food's contact with your mucosal lining.

Your GI tract is a long, windy road through your body, and it is covered in this mucosal lining. The digestive tract shares this lining with the respiratory system, so what lines your intestines also lines your lungs. In many systems of health in both Eastern and Western traditions, the digestive system and the respiratory system are linked both physically and energetically and are even considered a single system. This is because anything that impacts the mucosal lining tends to impact both the GI tract and the respiratory system. I see this link in my practice frequently—for example, it's not uncommon for people with asthma to suffer from constipation.

The interaction between food and your mucosal lining is not as quick as the interaction between food and your kidneys. While the kidneys filter all your blood in just under an hour, it can take an average of fifty hours, or up to five days in some cases, from the time you eat food to the time you excrete food. That means food is in contact with your mucosal lining for a long time. Some people are more efficient at this than others. Women typically take longer to digest food than men, for example. I find that people experiencing weight loss plateaus, however, aren't digesting food as efficiently as they could be. Food is in contact with the mucosal lining longer than it should be, and that translates to more time for things to go wrong.

Think of the mucosal lining as a bouncer for your intestines and lungs. It decides who gets in, who gets out and who won't be coming in again. When you eat food, the micronutrients enter the bloodstream through the mucosal lining because it allows them through. The only way nutrients can get into your system is if you inhale them or consume them (unless they are injected) because the mucosal lining manages this interaction between gut, lungs and bloodstream. The mucosal lining also plays an active role in digestion, secreting enzymes to help you digest food and making a comfy home for friendly bacteria that also help with digestion as well as immune function.

When something goes wrong with the mucosal lining, however, all kinds of bad things can happen inside you. If the "bouncer" leaves the door open, food substances, especially proteins, can get into the bloodstream, where they shouldn't be, causing weird allergies and even autoimmune disease (this is called *leaky gut syndrome*). Allergens and pathogens can get into the GI tract, or into the lungs, where they shouldn't be, causing gastrointestinal or respiratory illness. A swanky club can turn into a dive bar without a vigilant bouncer, and your body can become a metabolic mess without a healthy and sound mucosal lining.

When this is a chronic issue, lasting over a two-to-three-week period, the body begins to respond by developing hard, solid, yellow fat, which often accumulates around the torso, causing a barrel-chested look or a large, solid bowling-ball belly. Sometimes the effect is like a heavy blanket of fat lying over the whole body. This isn't lumpy, bumpy, squishy cellulite fat. It is thick, hard yellow fat and can develop into hard rolls that don't jiggle and seem like they are a permanent structure in your body. Sometimes you will also see fat hanging over the pubic area. When your bra straps are suddenly too tight, or your pants are binding at the waistline, or your shirt feels tight in places it was never tight before, or you just feel thicker, slower, stiffer, and stagnant all over, this is a sign of mucosal lining dysfunction. You can look in the mirror at your usually refined features and suddenly feel like you look chubby all over. One of my female clients told me that since she gained weight, she worried she "looked like a dude".

When this is your internal situation, your digestion will often stop working correctly. Your body begins to build up toxins in the GI tract, and good bacteria become overwhelmed by pathogenic bacteria. Immune system function can get suppressed, and the production of enzymes that help digest food and access stored fat can slow down or stop. Finally, your body puts out a distress call: *Toxin overload! Don't burn fat! Store it, store it, store it!*

The body is designed to protect itself from toxins, and it has to store any excess toxins somewhere. What is supposed to happen is that fat-soluble toxins are processed and eliminated through the bowels. If your bowels are working smoothly, the body gets the message that everything is all right and there is no need to store fat. In fact, it's great to start burning it for energy. If you are suffering from backed-up bowels, this results in emergency storage of fat-soluble toxins. The decision to burn or store all depends on the integrity of the mucosal lining and the movement, or lack of movement, in the GI tract.

Mucosal lining dysfunction can also cause a backup in your respiratory system. You can begin to accumulate phlegm in your throat and lungs. Phlegm is a protection against invaders such as viruses, bacteria and allergens, which can slip in when your mucosal lining isn't on the job. We produce phlegm to surround these foreign substances and carry them out of the body. If your mucosal lining is producing phlegm, you will know it because not only will you feel congested, but you will see mucus in the bowels, and the toilet will look slick or oily. That is the signal that bad guys are down there causing trouble. You want them out. But it's not enough to get rid of the phlegm. Get rid of the mucosal lining problem and phlegm production will take care of itself.

The bottom line is that if your mucosal lining is malfunctioning, digestion and respiration can get all backed up, causing issues from stomach pains to joint pain, and your body can morph into something you don't even recognize. If you don't intervene, poor digestive function can eventually cause a serious weight loss plateau made of fat that is very hard to chisel through—at least with ordinary diets.

THE D-BURN: DIGESTIVE INTERVENTION

Five days focused on anything is incredibly powerful. Can you imagine being given an entire workweek to focus intensely on a given task, with all the support you need and everything in place? You will be astonished at what you can pull off in your body in just five days. In five days, you'll lose inches in your belly, butt, hips and thighs. You'll let go of belly bloat and dig into that heavy thickness of fat blanketing your body.

In less than a week, we can begin to access and digest historical fat—you know, the fat that's been hanging around on the backs of your thighs since the eighties? By honing and healing your digestive and respiratory systems, you will release fat through the bowels and flush it right out of your life. You've been stuck, but plateaus should be short-lived and soon forgotten. Give me five days and you're going to access yellow fat for fuel—and it's going to burn, baby, burn.

WHAT YOU WILL ACHIEVE ON THE D-BURN

The D-Burn targets your body's digestion and assimilation of foods by soothing and healing the mucosal lining. You are going to stimulate the right digestive enzymes to not only break down the food you eat but also digest and eliminate the excess fat you're carrying. On the D-Burn, you will focus on melting away the whole hip-belly-butt band around the body. You'll also clear out the lungs at the same time, for an all-over feeling of clarity and lightness. All the waste you've been holding on to will be quickly and efficiently processed and moved out. You could lose up to five pounds in five days doing this work. You will also:

- Promote healthy gut bacteria; this will reduce bloat and belly swelling. When bad guys get into your gut, your body starts storing fat. We're going to clear out the riffraff.
- Target yellow fat, which is the hard, dense fat that likes to cling to your belly and torso. You will help your body make the enzymes you need to break through this thick, difficult fat so your body can eliminate it.

- Speed up the elimination of broken-down fat. You'll do this by facilitating the action of the digestive system through targeted foods, herbs and spices, especially cooked vegetables, proteins, starches and special GI-activating cooked fruit, to get things moving along.
- Nourish the digestive system with intensive micronutrients from lemon, cucumber, pumpkin and chia seeds, cauliflower, green beans, asparagus and cabbage. These support breaking down food and breaking down fat.
- Strengthen and nourish the lungs with supportive micronutrients from cinnamon, licorice, peppermint and ginger, and other practices that encourage a deeper purging of toxins in the respiratory tract.

With the D-Burn, you will notice not only smoother digestion and fewer digestive issues, but you will banish bloat and have the ability to breathe more calmly and deeply. You'll also slim down noticeably as you reclaim your smaller silhouette and enjoy a surge in energy. And the scale? It's going to reflect a happier number.

WHY YOU WILL LOSE WEIGHT ON THE D-BURN

Clearing up gas, constipation and bloating can make you *feel* like you've dropped five pounds, but with the D-Burn, you will do much more for your body than just getting waste moving through it in a timely manner. When you consume food, your body breaks it down. As it touches the mucosal lining in your digestive tract, this should set off a chain reaction of events. The presence of food triggers your mucosal lining to excrete the appropriate enzymes for digestion and fat metabolism, and the good bacteria in your intestine should help digest and process your food. Your mucosal lining should absorb nutrients from your food and selectively release these nutrients into the bloodstream, and then the waste you don't use should move on out the back door (so to speak).

If this isn't working, your body has accumulated that heavy layer of thick fat because your mucosal lining is letting bad guys (such as toxins and food particles) in, and keeping good guys (such as nutrients and good gut bacteria) out. Digestive problems such as gas, bloating, constipation and diarrhoea are symptoms of this dysfunction. When you remedy that through intensive digestive support, your body will stop storing fat to hold toxins and start burning fat for fuel. Your body will be primed to use that fat and handle toxin excretion effectively and efficiently.

On the D-Burn, not only will you be encouraging the digestive tract to empty when it has been stagnant, but you will also be providing your body with everything it needs to digest the food properly, nourish your mucosal lining and repopulate your gut with beneficial bacteria.

This is why the D-Burn is one of my favourite ways to break through historical plateaus. If you've lost weight many times in your life and you always get stuck in the same spot, then try becoming a D-Burner, to finally blaze a trail right past that stubborn number on the scale that feels like such an old "friend". It is awesome for those who feel like they aren't really digesting or breaking down the foods they are eating.

Your body has many ways of crying for help. Gas, bloating, constipation, diarrhoea, cramping and indigestion are obvious calls for the D-Burn. So are viruses, colds and phlegm, as well as brain fog, immobility and inflexibility in both mind and body. When your body cannot process its own waste or excavate its own fat stores, it needs the D-Burn. It needs your help.

I will provide you with all the tools you need—your metaphorical blowtorch. We'll take care of that tired old fat, just you wait and see!

YOUR D-BURN PLAN: WHAT TO EXPECT

If your rumbling tummy and phlegmy lungs are calling to you, you need to know what to do, so let's talk about exactly what will happen if you choose to embark upon the D-Burn. You will be calming your mucosal lining, ramping up yellow fat burning and heating up your body to blast through your weight loss plateaus. Every tool, every medicinal food item, every component is crucial and essential. You need to support every part of this process for maximum weight loss, and all these tools work together, so missing a small part of the process can limit your progress. Don't leave anything out!

You will be eating five times every day, and every meal and snack is filling and satisfying, so you'll never feel deprived. Instead, you'll feel nourished and supported, and you'll see just how quickly your body starts working the way it's supposed to work again.

Let's take a closer look at each of the D-Burn components.

D-Burn Smoothie: Your D-Burn Smoothie, with pumpkin seeds, chia seeds, lemon, green apple, raw basil and cucumber, will set you on the right track every day. Its purpose is to promote the excretion of the digestive enzymes that will target and break down yellow fat.

D-Burn Tea: You will drink D-Burn Tea throughout the day, with breakfast, lunch and dinner. You'll love this sweet tea made with cinnamon, ginger, peppermint, licorice and flaxseeds. This tea's primary function is to stimulate the movement of the bowels. We are looking for one to three large, well-formed bowel movements throughout the day. You won't be running to the bathroom unexpectedly.

D-Burn Soup: You will eat this soup at least twice a day, as a morning and afternoon snack, plus any other time you want it. It is loaded with micronutrients that nurture, soothe and heal the mucosal lining, and it has a spicy kick, full of green veggies, tomatoes, cabbage and as much or as little jalapeño pepper as you like.

D-Burn Recipes: The D-Burn recipes are for you to use to make your lunches and dinners. They are all in the recipe chapter and they are each formulated with specific thermogenic combinations of foods, herbs and spices that liquefy hard yellow fat and deliver it to the bloodstream so it can be excreted out of the body. You'll enjoy delicious dishes that are easy to make, such as Lentil Chilli, Shepherd's Pie, Beef and Broccoli Bowl, and Fennel and Salmon.

Water: Water is essential for all D-Burns because it keeps the bowels hydrated so that all the newly released toxic elements and ancient historical fat can quickly move out the back door. A healthy mucosal lining must also stay well hydrated, so drink up!

D-Burn Success Boosters: These natural, holistic remedies from health systems all over the world are effective as catalysts for all the things we want to accomplish on the D-Burn. Each one does something a little different, but they all either promote or intensify enzyme production, accelerate healing in the mucosal lining throughout the body, or help the bowel to purge and eliminate. These Success Boosters are also designed to increase the blood flow deep within that heavy, embedded fat in order to deliver the micronutrients that will emulsify the fat and carry it into the bloodstream to be excreted. You'll get a complete explanation of all the D-Burn Success Boosters and how to do them in Chapter 8.

GET YOUR CALENDAR

It's time to make a commitment and make it official. Put your five days down on your calendar right now so you can commit to them and schedule other commitments accordingly. You must hold these five days sacred and do all the components in order to effect real change in your digestive and respiratory system and break through your weight loss plateau. Make the D-Burn your priority.

So what do you think? Is the D-Burn for you? Read the next chapter to see whether the H-Burn will be even more beneficial for you right now. Or, if you know and are already sure that the D-Burn is it, go to Chapter 6 and get started right now.

CHAPTER FOUR

Are Hormones Causing Your Weight Loss Resistance?

Have a seat and tell me about your hormones. I don't expect you to know all about them on a biochemical level, but you probably already have some idea that hormones might be causing some of your issues, such as sudden weight gain and mood swings.

If you were my client, we would delve into all these issues and I would want to hear all about them because to me, they are significant red flags signalling that you need the H-Burn. This is just what happened with a former client of mine, whom I hadn't seen in seventeen years.

Delilah lives in Sacramento now, but she used to come up to my Colorado clinic regularly. She'd seen me on television when I was launching my first book, and this prompted her to reconnect by sending me an e-mail. She needed me again, she said. She wanted to see if I could create a quick programme for her to get eight to ten pounds off fast. Her motivation: a hiking tour with a group of cousins, up Machu Picchu.

High elevation and a heavy pack—at sixty years old, she wasn't sure she would have the strength and athleticism to keep up, especially as she had just gone through menopause and was suffering from a sudden jump in weight, insomnia and hot flushes she had hoped would stop after her periods stopped. No such luck. But could she really climb a mountain with hot flushes and that extra weight that equalled more than her pack?

Fortunately, we had just enough time to put her on the H-Burn, which was clearly the plan she needed. I gave her the recipes and told her to make big batches of H-Burn Tea and H-Burn Soup to take her through the ten days, which would end right before her trip began.

Delilah took my prescription seriously. She took on the plan like she was in training (which she was) and in ten days, she dropped ten pounds and her hot flushes stopped. She marched right up that mountain and she sent me a photo from what looked like the top of the world—and she looked ten years younger.

Maybe you need the same prescription. The third and final splinter that might be causing your stubborn weight loss resistance and keeping you from realizing the body you want is hormonal imbalance, and it can cause all the stereotypical symptoms you expect, plus more that you might never have guessed were related to your hormones. This is because hormones influence almost everything about how your body works. The micronutrients in the foods you eat go through a long and complex process in order to facilitate the creation and excretion of the hormones you need, but this process is vital for a healthy metabolism, as well as a functioning system that can get rid of excess fat the way it should.

There are many steps along the way, from eating food to maintaining a balance between the production and biosynthesis of hormones. The food you eat contains micronutrients that your body must convert into a usable form to make hormones. It also contains other micronutrients that your body uses to synthesize hormones for its needs and functions. This is incredibly important because hormones affect just about everything about you—how you move, perform, even how you feel. Hormones direct your hair growth, alter your skin quality and cause fluctuations in your energy and mood. They build muscle, make your heart beat and orchestrate the entire symphony that is you. They also have significant influence over when and how your body stores fat, and when and how your body decides to burn it for fuel. When any of the steps goes awry, the result is often hormone-based weight gain, because fat storage is one of the first lines of defence against hormonal imbalance. And there is nothing—I mean *nothing*—that will strand you on a plateau or cause weight loss resistance like hormone-based weight gain.

Let's take a closer look at how you are feeling and what signs and symptoms you might be experiencing, to determine whether you need the H-Burn.

SIGNS YOU NEED THE H-BURN

Let's consider whether your hormones are your biggest problem right now. Check all that apply to you:

- ❑ Is your hair dry and "crispy"?
- ❑ Are you losing hair at the crown of your head, or growing it in weird places, like on your chin?
- ❑ Are your heels cracked and dry?
- ❑ Is your skin crêpey and hanging off your cheeks or chin? Do you feel like you are losing collagen or elastin?
- ❑ Have you developed a muffin top and/or chubby knees?
- ❑ Is fat accumulating in places you never had it before? Do your clothes fit strangely now because of your changing body shape?
- ❑ Has your weight gain been rapid and then refused to budge?
- ❑ Is your libido MIA?
- ❑ If you are a woman, are your periods irregular? Is your PMS worse than normal? Are you having hot flushes or other menopausal symptoms?
- ❑ If you are a man, have you been diagnosed with low testosterone levels, or do you notice low energy and a diminished libido?
- ❑ Has your doctor told you that you have low vitamin D levels, even though you get plenty of sun? Do you also have low ferritin levels?
- ❑ Have you been experiencing an afternoon slump or sugar cravings around 3:00 to 4:00 p.m.?
- ❑ Are you eating a lot of sugar or simple carbs such as flour-based and sugar-based foods, then feeling great for a while but crashing later and feeling like you need a nap?
- ❑ Are you feeling moody, irritable or weepy? Do your moods feel unstable or unpredictable?

- Is your cholesterol high?
- Have you been diagnosed with hypoglycaemia, metabolic syndrome or Syndrome X, or has your doctor said you are prediabetic?
- Do you feel like you are out of step with your own life? Have you lost your natural rhythm?

If you checked more than half of these, then you need the H-Burn plan. If you checked almost all of them, then you have no time to lose. You need the H-Burn *stat*.

When you have hormonal imbalance, hormones are the reason why your body has changed shape and why you've developed fat in places you never had it before. The H-Burn is the best way to break through the most stubborn of plateaus: those caused by hormonal imbalance. This ten-day plan is more of a commitment than either the I-Burn or the D-Burn, but the results are stunning. You can get back the body you had before, or an even better one. Your skin will tighten up and get smoother and younger looking. Your moods will stabilize and you'll feel great. And all that lumpy white fat? With the H-Burn, you will incinerate your hormone-related weight-loss-limiting factors and your plateau will become a distant memory.

Another good reason to consider the H-Burn is when you have blood sugar issues (such as metabolic syndrome or Syndrome X). The liver regulates the glycogen, or sugar, in the body, and although the pancreas produces insulin, blood sugar issues are often an indication that the liver isn't processing and storing sugars as well as it should be. When blood sugar becomes elevated, the body begins to store that extra circulating sugar by producing more fat cells, and these are stubborn ones that don't want to go away.

Consider the H-Burn if you have low vitamin D levels, which indicate hormone imbalance. The liver is supposed to store vitamin D, and this vitamin, which is a precursor for hormones, is essential for activating all hormone receptor sites. If you don't have enough, there is a reason. Something isn't working correctly. It's common to be vitamin D deficient in cold climates or places with limited sun, but if you are fair skinned and live in Southern California or Florida and you're still vitamin-D deficient (I like to see levels above 50), give the H-Burn a try, even before you supplement with vitamin D. Test again after the ten days and see where you are. You might find your vitamin D levels have gone up into the normal range.

But measurable signs and symptoms aren't the only indications of hormone imbalance. Let's look at what's up with your roller-coaster emotions.

OTHER SIGNS YOU NEED THE H-BURN: YOUR MOOD

I often recommend the H-Burn for my clients who are struggling with certain kinds of emotional issues, and the most telltale signs are any kind of rhythmic disturbance or imbalance.

According to several ancient health systems, imbalance in the hormones mirrors imbalance in the emotions. If you have been feeling chronically indecisive, if you can't seem to come up with solutions to problems, if you notice you are more forgetful or you are feeling generally ineffective, this can be a sign of stagnation in the liver, gallbladder and thyroid, and the hormone imbalance that results from this. Hormones are all about rhythms, so if you feel out of sync with others or out of step with life, that can point to a hormonal issue.

Other signs are a general feeling of instability and moodiness. Not only are you making mountains out of fat, but you may be making mountains out of molehills in your personal life. This is different from the immediate and specific reactivity that characterizes mood signs on the I-Burn. This is more a generalized instability—moods that go up and down for no apparent reason: highs and lows, depression and anxiety, laughter followed by tears, or an inability to break out of an anxious or blue feeling, like a broken record that has lost the rhythm of its music. Moodiness is a key trait of someone who needs the H-Burn. If you are getting mood swings and displaying the good, the bad and the ugly, all within the span of about a minute; if you are feeling quick-tempered and aggressive; if you are prone to sudden bouts of road rage or you are throwing things and you're not standing on a pitcher's mound, then you need to be an H-Burner.

IS HORMONAL IMBALANCE CAUSING YOUR WEIGHT LOSS RESISTANCE?

I could write a whole book on hormones, but instead, let's just look briefly at what's going on in your body if you have hormonal imbalance.

When it works, hormonal balance is so complex and beautiful that it almost seems like magic, but when it goes badly, it can feel like you've got a curse on your head (or on your hips) that makes weight loss seem impossible. That's because without the hormones to direct the liquefication of body fat for fuel, your body only knows to hold on to those precious energy stores. And it holds on tight. As your hormones become increasingly imbalanced—either too much or too little of any or all of your hormones—your body becomes increasingly weight loss resistant. You can be eating all kinds of great food and it won't matter. What you eat will be a moot point because you can't access those nutrients. If the process of assimilating micronutrients in order to effect hormone balance isn't happening, then nothing is happening. And that means weight loss isn't happening either. You can juice, you can cleanse, you can diet all day long, but you have to be able to create the right balance of hormones in your body to regain your health and get your weight loss started again, and that takes a specific type of intervention.

What causes your hormones to go awry? Chronic stress is one of the most common reasons. Lack of sleep is another. Chronic exposure to toxins and the build-up of toxins in the body can tip hormones out of balance. You could ingest heavy metals through seafood, contaminated water, fractured dental fillings, or tainted health supplements. (I'm all about supplements, but not if they poison you!) Plastics can enter your system through Teflon cookware, plastic wrap, plastic water bottles and food storage containers, especially if you heat food in them. Heavy metals and plastics both can mimic hormones in the body, binding and gumming up hormone receptor sites, so the real hormones can't work.

Even viruses can interfere with hormone balance. Clinically, whenever I see someone with low vitamin D and ferritin levels (ferritin is a liver enzyme), I always suspect Epstein-Barr virus or cytomegalovirus. Both have been linked to disorders such as chronic fatigue and fibromyalgia, but more and more we're seeing that they impact the hormonal system. Vitamin D is stored in the liver, but these viruses inhibit the liver's ability to store vitamin D, especially in the presence of low ferritin levels. Also, elevated sustained antibodies to these viruses seem to inhibit weight loss, blocking the metabolic pathways for hormone metabolism.

Low vitamin D is not only a sign that you could have a virus but can be its own hormone-related issue. When I see low vitamin D in someone who gets enough sun (who lives, for example, in a warm sunny climate like Florida or California), I suspect hormone problems. Vitamin D is a fat-soluble hormone precursor, directly related to hormone metabolism. If you don't have adequate levels, this can inhibit the biosynthesis of the hormones you are producing, making hormonal imbalance even more profound.

Then there are hormone-based events that come with age, such as puberty, pregnancy, PMS, perimenopause (which can begin as early as the late thirties to early forties), menopause and postmenopause. Each of these events is characterized by hormonal changes that can cause a complex cascade of unpleasant symptoms. Men are not immune, either. "Manopause" is the unofficial term for hormonal changes in men that affect them physically and emotionally. There has been more and more research about the complexity of men's hormones. What we once thought was just about low testosterone, we now know also has to do with more complex processes, such as testosterone receptor sites being blocked and liver enzymes converting nonbioavailable testosterone into oestrogen. Signs of "manopause" include low testosterone levels, elevated oestradiol (a predominantly female hormone that men also have in lower amounts) and other symptoms similar to those that women experience during perimenopause, including reduction in adiponectin (a protein that regulates fat metabolism and glucose levels) and leptin resistance (resistance to the protein that helps regulate hunger and fat storage). Men can experience symptoms of "manopause" as early as their late thirties and early forties.

If you identify with hormonal changes and the havoc they wreak on your body and emotions, then the H-Burn is for you. It is designed to bring relief and balance to the chaos you are currently in.

Hormone imbalance can also be more pronounced in certain people, including those with polycystic ovarian syndrome (PCOS). PCOS is a condition that causes cysts to develop on the ovaries, along with high levels of male hormones in women, causing infertility, excessive hair growth, a higher risk for diabetes and other problems. Hormonal imbalance is also common in people who were extremely athletic during puberty, when all those oestrogen and testosterone pathways were awakening. When those people get older, come out of their growth phase and naturally settle down into more sedentary lifestyles in their thirties and forties, hormone-based weight gain is extremely common. This can be disheartening for people who were at the peak of their game just a few years before. Clients tell me, "But I won the state cup for soccer!", or "I was a champion swimmer!", or "I was captain of my football team. What's happening to my body!?"

The first signs of a hormonal problem include deep, emotional mood swings, not necessary surface-level reactivity to situations but finding yourself in high highs and low lows. Increased PMS and menopausal symptoms in women, sugar processing issues such as hypoglycaemia and even diabetes (insulin is a hormone), cravings, weird hair growth such as chin and moustache hair on women or losing hair on the crown of the head, even straightening of the pubic hair, and aggressive weight gain are all signs that hormones are either not being made, being made in excess, or being made but not being synthesized by your body so you can use them. Eventually, these problems may turn into insulin resistance, diabetes, serious mood issues such as depression and anxiety, and a major, noticeable accumulation of body fat. This makes the problem even worse, because fat itself produces even more dysfunctional hormones, compounding the problem.

People are often surprised to learn that fat produces hormones, but when fat cells take on a life of their own and begin this process, edging out the endocrine system like a bully, then the whole system can begin to misfire. Fat production becomes aggressive. The body begins to store fat in large areas very quickly. This causes even more of an imbalance in the hormones that normally work well together. Some hormone levels will get too high, and some will fall too low. You can develop problems with insulin secretion, causing blood sugar issues. You can pump out too much cortisol, the "stress hormone", causing insomnia, exhaustion, depressed immunity and anxiety. Or you could produce too much aldosterone, a hormone that regulates the balance of water and salt in your body and also regulates blood sugar. This can increase your blood pressure and cause the body to scavenge muscle for sugar in the form of glycogen, which can result in loss of muscle tone and loose saggy skin. If you've looked in the mirror and wondered, "Whose skin is this?" then you know what I mean. It droops and becomes crêpey and old-looking. Hormone-influenced body fat usually collects around the rib cage. You might notice lumps like a second set of breasts in weird places, such as under your bra line or on your upper back. You might develop saddlebags on the outsides of your thighs. Your ankles will get "fluffy", not with fluid but with fat, and you can get a muffin top—not from swelling as with inflammation, but from fat. It's not bloating; it's not water retention; it isn't even subcutaneous fat. It's deeper fat. It's puffy, fluffy fat that looks like it's there to stay. Your neck thickens and becomes creased, and your knees and calves get chubby, making your lower legs look thicker than usual.

All of this is white fat. It's fluffy and gelatinous and stubborn. You get rounder and lumpier, but most noticeably, your shape changes because fat accumulates unevenly. This is what is going on with my clients when they tell me they are getting fat in places they never got fat before. One client told me, "Yes, my butt is big, but I've always had a tiny waist. What happened to my waist?" Another told me, "Sure, I always carry a little weight in my belly, but where did these saddlebags come from? I've never had those before." And another: "I have wide hips but I've always had a flat belly. Whose stomach is this?"

The only way to intervene is to correct hormonal imbalance by restoring the body's micronutrient transformation function, thereby restoring an internal environment where hormones can be produced and synthesized correctly, and switching the body's fat-burning mechanism back on. As you begin to incinerate hormone-induced fat, your endocrine system can begin to restore homeostasis in its production and biosynthesis of hormones, taking the reins back from those rebel fat cells.

You can do this, even during the wild ride that is menopause. Hormonal changes associated with ageing do not mean you are doomed to become a metabolic mess and gain weight. You can take back the controls and restore your hormonal homeostasis. With further tweaking, your body can become a fat-burning machine, melting the strange lumps and sculpting your body into the shape you desire. Believe it or not, menopause can be a life change that feels natural and positive, rather than horrible. The H-Burn is your ticket.

THE H-BURN: HORMONAL INTERVENTION

If all of this speaks to you loud and clear, then get ready for an extreme transformation. If you are going to give me the luxury of a full ten days, then I can promise you some serious intervention focused on your hormonal system. We do this by working intensely on the liver, gallbladder and thyroid. The reason we do this is that these are the key areas that produce and synthesize hormones. Instead of just fixing the hormone imbalances themselves, we are going to repair the whole system that balances and synthesizes all your hormones. This supports the work of living that your body does every day, and it will correct hormone imbalance where it starts. There will always be times when your hormones fluctuate—times when you have more oestrogen, or less oestrogen, or more or less testosterone. Hormone balancing does not happen during a moment in time. It is a process, and as an H-Burner, you are going to nourish the organs and glands that produce and regulate hormones, so that you can be balanced going forward. When stress hits your life, when toxins hit your system, or when you go through natural hormone fluctuations, your body will be strong enough and balanced enough to handle it.

WHAT YOU WILL ACHIEVE ON THE H-BURN

On the H-Burn, you will target your body's transformation of food into hormones by facilitating the work of the liver, gallbladder and thyroid. Remember, we can't just target a given hormone. We have to target the whole hormone-balancing system, and this begins with the liver because the liver is what makes every hormone that is excreted from every gland in your endocrine system—your uterus, ovaries, testicles, pituitary, hypothalamus, thymus, pineal gland, adrenal glands and even your fat cells—active and bioavailable. If the liver says it's so, then it's so. If the liver doesn't say so, then it ain't happening. If you are in the throes of menopause and you are barely producing a teeny bit of oestrogen, the liver decides whether that oestrogen is effective or not. If you have low testosterone, the liver decides whether that testosterone is going to do you any good, and it also decides whether it will help the body produce more. The liver is powerful, and it waves the magic wand over your glands, directing the whole hormonal show. And the liver is extremely food-dependent. Of all the organs in the body, the liver is the one most impacted by what you eat.

The gallbladder and the thyroid are just as important as the liver. The gallbladder and the liver work together to emulsify fat. (Don't worry if you've had your gallbladder removed—in the absence of the gallbladder, the liver and the pancreas take over the gallbladder's former function.) The thyroid is a superhero gland that really is the anchor for the feedback loop for many of the hormones. The thyroid produces hormones that become bioactive in the liver and then adhere to receptor sites triggering the pituitary to communicate to the adrenals, the ovaries or the testicles. Even if you are on thyroid medication, you still need healthy receptor sites to take in the synthetic hormones. The production and biosynthesis of thyroid hormones triggers and determines the production and biosynthesis of hormones produced by all the other glands in the endocrine system—the ovaries, testicles, pituitary, adrenals and fat cells. When the metabolism is working well, it's because the thyroid says so.

You will strategically and intensively restore all the keepers of balance in your body on the H-Burn, so that when you are finished with the H-Burn, your body can go on stabilizing and strengthening your natural hormone regulatory system. Ten days means some heavy lifting, but it also means remarkable results. Get ready for fat to melt and fall off as your entire body changes shape. Your energy will soar and you will feel reborn. In ten days, you'll feel like you have a whole new body, and you could lose up to ten pounds! You will also:

- Deeply nourish the liver, gallbladder and thyroid with micronutrients from foods like grapefruit, coconut oil, dandelion root and parsley.
- Nourish the entire endocrine system with intensive micronutrients that support the proper production and regulation of hormones, with foods such as sunflower seeds, milk thistle, mushrooms and whole eggs.
- Target white fat, which is the lumpy, jiggly, tenacious fat that likes to accumulate in large amounts and in strange places, throwing your body shape out of proportion.
- Emulsify and release fat by using thermogenic combinations of

food, herbs, spices and teas that ferret out and dissolve hormone-induced fat, such as turmeric, ginger, black pepper and crushed red pepper flakes as well as coconut oil, coconut milk and avocado.

- Stabilize the emotional symptoms so common with imbalanced hormones, including moodiness, irritability, aggressiveness, anxiety and depression.
- Deluge the body with healthy fat, to stimulate fat metabolism and to repair dry, cracked, crêpey skin, splitting nails and strawlike hair.

With the H-Burn, you will attack stubborn white hormone-induced fat, stabilize your body's hormonal balance, and soothe your mood while you smooth your new and unwelcome bulges and jiggles. You will bust through your most stubborn weight loss plateau and watch the number on the scale start plummeting downward.

So You Have Thyroid Issues?

If you have thyroid issues, you may be wondering whether the H-Burn is appropriate for you, or if you need to make any changes to it. Whether you've been diagnosed with hyperthyroidism, Hashimoto's disease, Graves' disease, had your thyroid removed or are on thyroid medication, you are in the right place. The thyroid is one of the primary regulators of the entire hormone system throughout your body. Any thyroid-related imbalance, including any disease process, requires strategic nurturing in order to create homeostasis in the hormones that affect the metabolism. The H-Burn is exactly the place for that strategic nurturing. If thyroid issues are your issues, then stop whatever you are doing right now and schedule your H-Burn!

WHY YOU WILL LOSE WEIGHT ON THE H-BURN

The H-Burn targets fat intensely because of how closely hormones and fat work together. Hormone receptor sites are active and working, and they send out a siren song to the hormones: *Come to me, hormones!* But when they aren't working, then the hormones don't know where to go. They just keep circulating throughout the body, like ships without a home port. When the body senses all those circulating hormones, it calls out to the fat cells for help: *What are we going to do about all these hormones?*

Unfortunately, this is like asking that guy who got kicked out of basic maths to teach a college maths class. Fat cells can create hormones too, but when they suddenly start acting as part of the endocrine system, like a secondary gland, they tend to cause a lot of trouble. Fat cells start creating their own hormones, which tend to intensify sugar cravings, disrupt the production of hormones that make you feel stable and good (such as endorphins and dopamine) and inhibit serotonin receptor sites, which can cause problems like depression and ramp up fat production even more—because why not bring along more friends? Soon, the endocrine system can become completely overwhelmed and hormone levels get further and further out of whack.

The liver is important in this process because it directs sugar in the blood either into the liver, for storage, or into the muscles, for energy and repair, or in the case of too much sugar, into fat cells, for later use. When the liver becomes overwhelmed, malnourished or too clogged with fat, it may slack off on this job, and blood sugar can remain circulating in the blood. This can cause an excess of insulin production, and when this process goes on for too long, this can cause insulin resistance, metabolic syndrome, even diabetes. Intensive micronutrient support to the liver gives it the resources it needs to take its proper active role in directing blood sugar into the right places. The support you will give your gallbladder on the H-Burn plan is similarly conducive to rapid fat loss because the gallbladder (as well as the liver) produces bile, which is the catalyst for emulsifying that lumpy white fat you are so tired of lugging around.

The thyroid governs production of all the other hormones. It is the master hormone regulator, and it needs its own nurturing in order to direct proper hormone balance. This will keep the body in a calm state rather than in a state of crisis, where it is more likely to cling to fat just in case it might be needed for reserve energy.

Finally, the rapid incineration of fat you will accomplish on the H-Burn will keep fat from interloping into the job of the endocrine system. Fat cells can't produce trouble making excessive hormones if you've burned them off! This is like kicking the unqualified teachers out of the classroom and replacing them with proper professors (i.e., the glands that are supposed to be producing hormones will have what they need to get back to work).

YOUR H-BURN PLAN: WHAT TO EXPECT

All right already, mood swings, we hear you! Now that you've got yourself pegged as someone who is in need of the H-Burn, let's talk about what's going to happen over the next ten days. Every part of the H-Burn is crucial for accomplishing specific jobs in your body: fat incineration, liver support, gallbladder support, thyroid support, hormone regulation and mood stabilization. You're going to feel and look better than you have in a long time in just about ten days from now, but the H-Burn's effectiveness will be diminished with every missing tool. Every item on this list is required. Don't skip the smoothie. Don't ditch the tea. Eat all your soup, and adhere to your H-Burn food list like it is gospel. You must include every element, including the requisite amount of daily water and the required number of Success Boosters, if you want to make the kind of dramatic impact that is the inevitable result of this process. Follow the rules, and you'll barely recognize yourself in ten days.

You'll get to eat five times every day so you won't feel hungry, but you will be feeling more stable as you burn fat and get your hormones back into good working order.

Now let's take a closer look at each of the parts so essential to H-Burn success.

> **H-Burn Smoothie:** Your H-Burn Smoothie stimulates the enzymes in the blood that proteolyze (or break down) fat by stimulating and supporting bile production in the gallbladder and liver through the actions of the grapefruit, beetroot, kale, spinach, coconut oil and sunflower seeds.

> **H-Burn Tea:** This tea is highly targeted to nurture the thyroid, which sends so many crucial messages to your hormones and other glands. It contains micronutrients found in limes, milk thistle, dandelion root and turmeric to support the liver and thyroid and im-

prove thyroid hormone activation, as well as clearing receptor sites so that released hormones can more effectively convert into their active forms and help you get on with the business of living.

H-Burn Soup: H-Burn Soup contains a specific thermogenic combination of micronutrients from garlic, mushrooms, parsley, onions and green vegetables that feed the liver so that it can be more effective in converting secreted hormones into active hormones.

H-Burn Recipes: The specific foods, herbs, spices and recipes feed and stimulate the liver and gallbladder, increasing the fat-emulsifying effects as well as stabilizing hormone regulation. The proteins on this plan also feed the liver, which needs amino acids created from proteins to function correctly, and the fats will help your body slip into fat-burning mode. These foods nurture the thyroid and stimulate the healthy activation of thyroid receptor sites. Best of all, they are delicious—you'll get to enjoy meals such as Herbed Egg Salad, Chicken Avocado Salad with Creamy Coconut-Mango Dressing, Stuffed Cabbage Rolls with Wild Mushroom Sauce, Rosemary Chicken with Roasted Veggies, and Greek-Style Baked Cod with Artichokes.

Water: Water is important for H-Burns because of the duration and effectiveness of this plan. Because of the intense level of fat burning, fat-soluble toxins will be released in a steady stream into your bloodstream, and you need to flush them out so you don't reabsorb them or suffer uncomfortable symptoms. The only way to do this efficiently is with significant hydration. This hydrates the bowels to keep you flushing regularly and sufficiently. Hydration is extremely important in this plan since a lot of toxins will be released. This is why you'll be drinking half your body weight in ounces of water every day.

H-Burn Success Boosters: Each and every H-Burn Success Booster is a catalyst for one or more of the intensive actions happening in the body during the next ten days. Please do as many as you can! Remember, we are not supporting the hormones directly. We are cultivating the system that produces and manages hormones, and hormones are relevant to *everything you do.* H-Burn Success Boosters, including exercises that cycle between cardio, weight lifting and relaxation, shift and establish a rhythm to mimic what you want your hormones to do in the body. This can make a major impact not just on your weight loss but on your entire life. They are important for increasing health, longevity, a positive mood and energy, and of course, they are a huge catalyst for weight loss. I hope these particular Success Boosters will play a vital role in your life even after you are finished with the H-Burn.

GET YOUR CALENDAR

Committing to a plan for ten days is a lot bigger deal than committing to a plan for just three days, but these ten days are crucial, so I want you to get your calendar, mark those days, and keep them sacred. This is no time to be partying, going out to fancy restaurants, drinking alcohol or cheating with junk food. Adhere to all aspects of the plan if you want the intensive and dramatic hormone-balancing results. Choose a ten-day period where you don't have a lot of social obligations.

If you are especially interested in easing PMS symptoms that you tend to get during the week before your period, start the H-Burn on the third day of your period. The reason for this is that how you support your body in the first fourteen days of your cycle is what determines how your body will react in the next cycle. Day three in particular is when your body makes a hormonal shift between oestrogen and progesterone. If you start the H-Burn on day three and continue through day thirteen, then you should notice that the next month, your PMS will be significantly reduced. You may notice fewer mood swings and other PMS symptoms such as acne, irritable bowel symptoms, tender breasts, back pain and headaches.

PART TWO

THE BURN

CHAPTER FIVE

I-Burn: Inflammation Intervention

It's time to access the strength, determination and fire you need to overcome your obstacles, and you're going to do it with the I-Burn. You're going to banish the swelling, water, and subcutaneous fat to reclaim your natural shape. You're my I-Burner now, so let's get ready to turn up the heat.

READY . . .

You will be most successful with the I-Burn if you are mentally prepared. Here is what you can expect over the next three days:

- You will eat breakfast within thirty minutes of waking every day. This is extremely important for the I-Burn because when you sleep, you are experiencing a period of rest and restoration. Your body is building bone, hair, skin and muscle, and repairing all your systems. As soon as you get up, the detoxification process begins and your body works quickly to reestablish a balanced pH and purge toxins from the night's work. With this, a process of inflammation can start in the body. The sooner you restore the body with micronutrients from breakfast, the sooner you help establish that balanced pH, stimulate anti-inflammatory action in the body and set the tone for the day.

- You will have one I-Burn Smoothie every day for breakfast, for a total of three over the course of the three days. Make these fresh, as you need them.

- You will have at least three cups of I-Burn Tea every day: one serving for breakfast, another for lunch, and a third for dinner, for a total of nine cups over the course of the three days. You will brew this ahead of time in one big batch. Just warm up the tea as you need it.

- You will have two servings of I-Burn Soup, one for lunch and one for dinner, every day (1 serving is 450g). You may have more than this, but this is the minimum. Generally, I tell my clients not to consume over four servings of soup per day. There is really no good reason to eat any more than that. You can make all the soup you need ahead of time, then warm it up as you need it.

- You will have two pieces of fruit per day for each of two snacks, for a total of six pieces of fruit over the three days. You can choose any fruit from the food list at the end of this chapter, but I have made specific suggestions for you in the meal map and in the day-by-day list.

- You will have lunch and dinner each day, for a total of three lunches and three dinners. Each will consist of a cup of I-Burn Tea, a serving of I-Burn Soup, and either an I-Burn Recipe, or a serving each of vegetables, protein and a healthy fat such as extra-virgin olive oil, avocado or pine nuts (all allowed foods are in the I-Burn food list at the end of this chapter). The recipes I suggest you make are listed on the meal map and within the day-by-day descriptions. The actual recipes are grouped near the back of the book for ease of access.

All lunch recipes serve one person, and all dinner recipes serve two people, unless otherwise indicated, such as when you will be saving half for another meal. When this is the case, I will alert you to set aside half the recipe for the freezer. I'll also prompt you about when to defrost this portion. If you want to serve more people for any meal or have leftovers, you can double or even triple the recipes, but factor this in by increasing the amount of appropriate ingredients on your grocery list.

If you team up with a roommate or family member and plan to double all recipes, you can have more fun and support on *The Burn*.

- You will be able to eat any food from the I-Burn's specific list of free foods whenever you want if you are ever hungry during the day. These are:

  - I-Burn Soup
  - I-Burn Tea
  - Celery
  - Cucumber
  - Jicama or Turnips
  - Lemons
  - Limes
  - Radishes

- You will drink half your body weight in ounces of water every day. I'll remind you throughout the day on your meal map and day-by-day schedule, but try to finish 25 per cent of your water by midmorning, 50 per cent by lunch, 75 per cent by dinner, and 100 per cent by bedtime. I prefer that you use high-quality spring water if you can. If this isn't possible, at least use some sort of purification or filtering system rather than plain tap water.

- You will do one Success Booster each day for the next three days. You get to choose which ones you want to try and when you want to try them, but I will give you some reminders and suggestions in the day-by-day plan. Look over the Success Booster options at the end of this chapter, and find detailed descriptions for how to do each one in Chapter 8, including what supplies you might need for any, so you can add these items to your shopping list.

- You will buy everything you need ahead of time. You may also prepare your tea, soup, lunches and dinners ahead of time, so all you have to do is take them out of the refrigerator and enjoy. (I suggest you make your I-Burn Smoothie fresh each morning, though.)

- This chapter includes a grocery list with everything you will be eating for the next three days. You may substitute any foods you can't or don't like to eat with items from the same list (vegetable for vegetable, fruit for fruit, protein for protein). Don't forget to add whatever you will need for the Success Boosters you choose.

Now it's time to jump in and get everything ready. Let's start with your grocery list.

I-BURN GROCERY LIST

You probably already have some of these things, so scour your refrigerator, freezer and pantry to determine what you have and what you still need. Note that this list tells you exactly how much you will need of something, so you can decide for yourself what size package, bottle or bag to buy, or whether you already have enough of something at home. Also consider that in many health food stores, you can buy in bulk and will be able to purchase exact amounts. If you have access to bulk foods, you can even bring your measuring cups and spoons to the store with you. When you have the option and it is affordable, always choose organic.

Also, a reminder: if there is any food that you do not like or cannot eat, or that is not available or in season for you, you can substitute it for another food within the same category on the food list at the end of this chapter. Again: fruit for fruit, vegetable for vegetable, protein for protein.

PORTION GUIDELINES

A special note about portion sizes: the portions for the recipes and the foods on the food lists are for anyone, man or woman, no matter how much weight you need to lose. Some people ask me about protein. All protein serving sizes are 110g for meat or poultry and 175g for seafood or fish. Do you need more if you are a man, or if you have more weight to lose? Actually, all you need is enough protein to provide the building blocks for repair, and this amount is perfectly sufficient for anyone. If you feel like you need more food, remember that you can always have unlimited soup, tea and free foods. Fill up on soup and tea because they are powerful sources of repair. And don't forget your water!

Free Foods

I-Burn Soup
I-Burn Tea
Celery
Cucumber

Jicama/Turnips
Lemons
Limes
Radishes

Vegetables

1 small carton alfalfa sprouts
700g beetroots
2 heads green or red cabbage
7 carrots
4 celery stalks with leaves
450g spring greens, chard and/or
    dandelion leaves
2 cucumbers
1 daikon or white radish, root
    and top (if tops are available),
    enough for 225g chopped
8 garlic cloves
2 large jicama/turnips

225g shiitake or maitake
    mushrooms, fresh or dried
225g white button
    mushrooms
1 large red onion
2 root vegetables: turnips,
    parsnips and/or swede
    (about 400g diced)
2 sweet potatoes
1.35kg fresh spinach
3 tomatoes
7 courgettes

Fruit

2 avocados
250g blueberries (fresh or
    frozen)
180g cranberries (fresh or
    frozen)

10 lemons
8 limes
3 pears
1 pink grapefruit
300g diced watermelon

Protein

60g black beans (preferably
    sprouted, but not required)
175–275g Dover sole fillet (or any
    light wild-caught fish)
2 tablespoons hummus

50g raw pine nuts (or replace
    with walnuts)
175g tinned sardines
125g raw walnuts (or 190g if not
    using pine nuts)

Herbs, spices, sweeteners and miscellaneous

½ teaspoon cayenne pepper
3 tablespoons celery seed

Dash of ground cinnamon
1 bunch fresh coriander or parsley

8 tablespoons extra-virgin olive
   oil

Dash of ground nutmeg

9 tablespoons dried parsley

Sea salt

Optional for sweetening: birch
   xylitol or pure stevia

SET . . .

Now that you have the ingredients you need, it's time to do your recipe prep. Please don't skip this and think you will just make everything as you need it. This is extremely important for your plan to go smoothly. I often make my I-Burn Smoothie each morning, but you should prepare your I-Burn Tea and Soup *before you start*. Some of my clients also like to make some or even all of their lunches or dinners, so everything is assembled and ready to enjoy straight out of the refrigerator or is easy to just warm up. It's only three days, so everything you make will stay fresh. Store everything in the refrigerator in easily accessible containers, so all you have to do when you start is measure out your portion and enjoy.

I-BURN TEA POWER

Every ingredient in this tea has a specific function for what we are trying to accomplish on this three-day plan:

- Lemon juice helps balance pH, making you more alkaline. It is also rich in vitamin C and can help the pancreas balance insulin, so it inhibits insulin resistance.

- Lemon peel contains bioflavonoids, which are naturally anti-inflammatory. These are released from the peel with boiling.

- Celery seed has antibacterial properties and has traditionally been used for urinary tract disorders, but for you, it can help combat any low-grade infections you might have. It also has diuretic properties so it can help flush out old fluid that has been sitting around in your face, hands and ankles.

- Parsley contains unusual but powerful compounds: a volatile oil containing myristicin, limonene, eugenol and alpha-thujene, which are natural diuretics and also lower cortisol (the stress hormone) and help shuttle fat out of the fat cells. It also has apiin, apigenin, chrysoeriol and luteolin. These reduce swelling and are catalysts for the metabolism of cellulite.

- Cayenne pepper increases blood flow into fat cells and increases body temperature. It also possesses enzymes that liquefy fat cells in hard-to-reach places.

Turn to Chapter 9 for all your recipes. Your core recipes for this three-day plan—I-Burn Smoothie, I-Burn Tea, and I-Burn Soup—are all in the recipe chapter. Make your tea and soup, and then scan through the other recipes to see what else you might want to make ahead. If you don't like a recipe, you can substitute any lunch or dinner recipe, but just make sure you have one serving each of vegetable, fruit, and protein for lunch and also for dinner. And be sure to adjust your grocery list accordingly.

This is also the time to choose your Success Booster. Some are easy, but the Success Boosters listed in the Intense Boosts section either need special equipment or are somewhat intense and may not be for everyone. For detailed descriptions on how to do each of these and what they will do for you, see Chapter 8. Look there for more information on the ones that interest you. And remember—one a day minimum. You can always do more!

I-BURN SUCCESS BOOSTERS

Exercise:
30-minute walk, preferably outdoors in a beautiful natural setting
Gentle yoga or stretching, 20 to 30 minutes or take a class

To Add to Your Smoothie:
225g kale or spinach

To Add to Your Tea:
1 dandelion tea bag

To Add to Your Soup:
225g chopped fresh beetroot greens

Easy Boosts:
Deep breathing

Epsom salts bath

Essential oil self-massage: fennel, cinnamon, clove, eucalyptus, bergamot, thyme, rose

Flower essences

Meditation

Reflexology

Targeted I-Burn supplement protocol

Intense Boosts:
Infrared sauna

Lymphatic massage

Rebounding

Choose which three or more you want to try, then flip to Chapter 8 to see what you need and what to do. Schedule these into your three days now. All your preparation efforts now will pay off when you embark upon your three-day campaign. Would you go to war without your weapons? Never! Have everything you need fully prepared and you will emerge victorious.

GO!

Your supplies are on hand. Your food is prepared. Your Success Boosters are chosen. Here are the next three days, all laid out for you. You've done all the prep, so now all you have to do is follow along. Of course, although I have designed your battle plan the same way I do for many of my clients, there is a lot about you I don't know. There may be certain foods you don't like or can't eat because you are allergic to or intolerant of them. That's fine. If you don't like broccoli, for example, look at the list and find another item in the vegetable list, and substitute it. Just don't substitute with something from another list. For example, you can substitute kale for broccoli, but you can't substitute blueberries for broccoli.

There are negotiables (which vegetable, which fruit, which Success Booster), and there are non-negotiables (you eat the requisite foods; you have your smoothie, tea and soup; you eat as often as I say; and you do I-Burn-approved Success Boosters). Follow the plan, but make it work for you.

I-BURN PLAN, DAY-BY-DAY

YOUR I-BURN TO-DO LIST

❑ Did I get all the necessary ingredients for the recipes I will make?

❑ Did I prepare 9 cups (or more) of I-Burn Tea to keep in the refrigerator?

❑ Did I prepare 6 servings (or more) of I-Burn Soup to keep in my refrigerator?

❑ If I'm using bottled water, do I have enough to drink half my body weight in ounces each day for the next three days?

❑ Do I know what my daily Success Boosters will be each day, and do I have everything I need for them?

I-Burn Daily Targets:

- Eat three meals and two snacks. Do not skip any of these, even if you aren't hungry.
- Drink half your body weight in ounces of water. No other beverages except I-Burn Tea are allowed.
- If you drink coffee or caffeinated tea, replace it with I-Burn Tea.
- Nosh on free foods or sip I-Burn Soup or I-Burn Tea between meals if you get hungry.
- Don't forget your daily I-Burn Success Booster.

I-BURN MEAL MAP

Here are your three days, at a glance. Snap a picture with your phone or make a copy and keep it with you so you always know what to eat.

DAY 1

BREAKFAST

SNACK

25%

1 pear

LUNCH

Spinach Avocado Salad with Watermelon

50%

SNACK

200g watermelon pieces

75%

DINNER

Dover Sole with Roasted Vegetables

100%

AT A GLANCE
- 1 smoothie
- 3 cups tea
- 2 servings soup
- 2 fruits
- Spinach Avocado Salad with Watermelon
- Dover Sole with Roasted Vegetables
- Half your body weight in ounces of water
- At least 1 Success Booster

DAY 2

BREAKFAST

SNACK

200g watermelon pieces 25%

LUNCH   Hummus Coleslaw 50%

SNACK

1 pear 75%

DINNER Roasted Vegetables on Courgette "Pasta" 100%

AT A GLANCE
- 1 smoothie
- 3 cups tea
- 2 servings soup
- 2 fruits
- Hummus Coleslaw
- Roasted Vegetables on Courgette "Pasta"
- Half your body weight in ounces of water
- At least 1 Success Booster

DAY 3

BREAKFAST

SNACK
1 pink grapefruit with cinnamon 25%

LUNCH Sardines and Cucumbers 50%

SNACK
75%
100g blueberries

DINNER   Mexican Dinner Salad
Cayenne Watermelon 100%

AT A GLANCE
- 1 smoothie
- 3 cups tea
- 2 servings soup
- 2 fruits
- Sardines and Cucumbers
- Mexican Dinner Salad
- Cayenne Watermelon
- Half your body weight in ounces of water
- At least 1 Success Booster

DAY 1

When You Wake Up:
- Weigh yourself. You won't be doing this again for three days. Use this number to calculate how much water you will drink every day for the next three days: half your body weight in ounces. If you don't have a scale and don't care about the numbers, don't worry about this. You probably know what you weigh from your last doctor visit. Figure your water consumption using that number.
- Plan your Success Booster for the day, and when you will do it. Maybe add 225g of kale to your morning smoothie?

Breakfast:
1 serving **I-Burn Smoothie**
1 cup **I-Burn Tea**

I-Burn Targeted Nutrition: Cranberries
Cranberries contain powerful anti-inflammatory phytonutrients called anthocyanins. They also contain the bioflavonoids called quercetin, myricetin, and kaempferol, which have natural anti-inflammatory and antihistamine properties. Use fresh or frozen. They are nutritionally equivalent.

Mid-morning Snack:
1 pear

Finish 25 per cent of your water.

Lunch:
1 cup **I-Burn Tea**
1 serving (450g) **I-Burn Soup**
1 serving **Spinach Avocado Salad with Watermelon**

If you do not want to make this recipe, you can also choose 1 portion each of vegetables, protein and a healthy fat from the food list at the end of this chapter, in addition to your I-Burn Tea and I-Burn Soup.

Finish 50 per cent of your water.

Afternoon:

Finish 75 per cent of your water. You probably won't be physically hungry, but if you are in the habit of overeating, drinking water can help distract you.

Afternoon Snack:

200g watermelon pieces

Dinner:

1 cup **I-Burn Tea**
1 serving (450g) **I-Burn Soup**
Dover Sole with Roasted Vegetables

As with lunch, if you have already decided not to use a recipe, you may choose 1 portion each of vegetables, protein and a healthy fat from the food list at the end of this chapter, in addition to your I-Burn Tea and I-Burn Soup.

Mushroom Power

I-Burn Soup is a vegetarian soup made with mushroom broth, and it will calm the inflammation and flush excess fluid from your body. The key is the mushrooms, which contain an antioxidant called *ergothioneine*. Scientists are just now beginning to recognize ergothioneine as a "master antioxidant". It is also an amino acid containing sulphur, which is great for your skin.

Evening:

Finish 100 per cent of your water.

Bedtime:

Go to bed in time to get eight hours of sleep, to keep your body working efficiently. This is also important for controlling stress hormones and gives the kidneys and lymphatic system plenty of time to integrate the nourishment and support you've provided them throughout the day. You might need to get up during the night to use the bathroom as your body continues to adjust to increased fluid intake. This is a good sign that your kidneys and bladder are clearing out the junk.

Kidneys and Salt

Table salt is one of the worst foods for the kidneys. From a Western medicine perspective, when an individual has kidney problems due to high blood pressure or kidney disease, doctors look closely at sodium consumption. We have adulterated our table salt to such an extent that it has become detrimental to kidney function and water exchange. In Chinese medicine, real, natural salt is nurturing for the kidneys. Look for Celtic sea salt or other true natural salts. Some are pink, green or grey and have flecks of minerals in them.

DAY 2

When You Wake Up:

- Measure out your water for the day—half your body weight in ounces—and start sipping. A squeeze of lemon juice in your water can help wake up your body and get you ready for breakfast.
- Schedule your Success Booster for the day. Maybe this is a good day to try deep breathing or meditation in the morning or after work.

Breakfast:

1 serving **I-Burn Smoothie**

1 cup **I-Burn Tea**

Mid-morning Snack:

200g watermelon pieces

Finish 25 per cent of your water.

Lunch:

1 cup **I-Burn Tea**

1 serving (450g) **I-Burn Soup**

Hummus Coleslaw

Finish 50 per cent of your water.

I-Burn Targeted Nutrition: Daikon

Daikon means "great root" in Japanese. It is also sometimes called white radish. Daikon is a common hangover remedy because it has strong diuretic and anti-inflammatory properties. One of these veggies has approximately 2 grams of alkalizing protein.

Afternoon:

Finish 75 per cent of your water.

Afternoon Snack:

1 pear

Dinner:

1 cup **I-Burn Tea**
1 serving (450g) **I-Burn Soup**
Roasted Vegetables on Courgette "Pasta"

Evening:

Finish 100 per cent of your water.

Bedtime:

Go to bed in time to get eight hours of sleep, to keep your body working efficiently. You should sleep well tonight—your body has spent about thirty-six hours detoxifying and you should be feeling clean and calm. You may already be adjusting to increased fluid intake, but if you need to use the bathroom during the night, again, remember that you are continuing to release all that fluid you've been storing. You'll be looking noticeably slimmer in the morning!

DAY 3

When You Wake Up:

- Measure out your water for the day—half your body weight in ounces—and start sipping. Think about continuing to drink this much water, even after you've conquered those three pounds and moved on. It's always a good idea to help your kidneys along with proper hydration, and most people don't drink enough water. Plan your Success Booster for the day. Maybe a nice relaxing Epsom salts bath tonight would be the perfect way to wrap up your I-Burn.

Breakfast:

1 serving **I-Burn Smoothie**

1 cup **I-Burn Tea**

Mid-morning Snack:

1 pink grapefruit with a sprinkle of cinnamon

Finish 25 per cent of your water.

Lunch:

1 cup **I-Burn Tea**

1 serving (450g) **I-Burn Soup**

1 serving **Sardines and Cucumbers**

Finish 50 per cent of your water.

Afternoon:

Finish 75 per cent of your water.

Afternoon Snack:

100g blueberries

Dinner:

1 cup **I-Burn Tea**

1 serving (450g) **I-Burn Soup**

1 serving **Mexican Dinner Salad**

1 serving **Cayenne Watermelon**

I-Burn Targeted Nutrition: Cayenne Pepper

Cayenne pepper contains a phytonutrient called capsaicin that is a powerful anti-inflammatory that supports lymphatic drainage and pH balance.

Evening:

Finish 100 per cent of your water.

Bedtime:

Just because the three days are over tomorrow doesn't mean you can start skimping on sleep again. This is a great habit to continue. And tomorrow morning? Your rings will be looser and you will notice your ankles are looking slimmer. Your skin will look radiant, tighter and younger, because you didn't just deflate your swelling, you nourished your entire system. Your circulation is good and your body isn't in panic mode anymore, holding on to every drop of water. Go ahead, wear that fitted dress tomorrow. You're going to rock it!

I-BURN OPTIONS

You may not be able to or want to eat every item on your I-Burn grocery list, but you can always substitute an item with another from the food list that follows. If you hate asparagus or watermelon is out of season or you would really rather do a sauna than meditate, we can totally make that work. You have options.

Here is your complete I-Burn food list. If it's not on the list or chosen as a Success Booster, then it is not in your toolbox, so forget about it.

I-Burn Food List

Free Foods

Eat as much as you want!

I-Burn Soup	Jicama/Turnips
I-Burn Tea	Lemons
Celery	Limes
Cucumber	Radishes

Vegetables (minimum serving size is 150g raw)

Alfalfa sprouts	Kelp
Artichoke and artichoke hearts	Mushrooms (baby bella, maitake,
Asparagus	portobello, shiitake, white
Beetroots, roots and tops (greens)	button)
Bell peppers (red)	Onions (red)
Brussels sprouts	Parsnips
Cabbage (red or green)	Radishes
Carrots	Rocket
Cauliflower	Seaweed
Celery	Spinach
Courgettes	Spirulina
Cucumbers	Spring greens
Daikon/white radish	Swede
Dandelion greens	Sweet potatoes
Garlic	Swiss chard
Ginger	Tomatoes
Green beans	Turnips
Hearts of palm	Watercress
Jicama/Turnips	Yams
Kale	

Fruits (serving size is 1 piece or 150g—you may use fresh or frozen fruit)

Asian pears	Grapefruit
Blueberries	Lemons
Cherries	Limes
Cranberries	Pears

Persimmons

Raspberries

Pineapple

Watermelon

Pomegranates

Proteins (serving size is 110g meat/poultry; 175g seafood/fish; 1 egg; 75g legumes; 225g grains; 50g nuts/seeds; 110g hummus)

Adzuki beans, sprouted

Black beans

Crab

Eggs

Fish, raw (such as sashimi)

Fish, white (such as Dover sole, cod, tilapia, halibut, or any white fish, preferably wild-caught)

Hummus

Kaniwa, sprouted (a small grainlike seed related to quinoa, sometimes called "baby quinoa")

Kidney beans

Lentils, sprouted

Mung beans

Oysters (in water or olive oil, or raw)

Pine nuts

Pumpkin seeds, raw, preferably sprouted

Quinoa, ideally sprouted or whole-grain

Sardines, tinned

Sesame seeds, black

Sunflower seeds, raw, preferably sprouted

Turkey

Walnuts, raw

Wild rice, sprouted

Fats (serving size is ¼ avocado or 1 to 2 tablespoons other fat or oil)

Avocado

Coconut butter, raw

Coconut milk

Olive oil, extra-virgin

Miscellaneous

Birch xylitol

Cayenne pepper

Celery seed

Cinnamon

Coriander, fresh

Nutmeg

Parsley, fresh or dried

Pepper, black

Red pepper flakes, crushed

Sea salt

Stevia, pure

YOU DID IT! NOW WHAT?

Congratulations! You did it! Three days and you are enjoying immense health benefits, especially in your kidneys. You should be feeling slimmer, tighter and more radiant, and I bet your skin looks fantastic. I hope you will go back to your regular routine, but maybe leave a few of your less-healthy habits behind. You've done it, it wasn't painless but it wasn't so bad, and now you've got another tool to keep in your back pocket. Pull it out whenever you need it.

Many of my clients continue to use the smoothies, teas and soups that they love, even when they aren't on the programme. Your kidneys are so important that it's always a good idea to use the foods that nurture and support them. Maybe you enjoyed the smoothie. Have it for breakfast often. Is the tea tasty? Make a big batch every week and sip on it frequently. If the soup makes you feel fantastic, keep it in the freezer for a quick lunch or dinner when you don't have time to cook and want hydration and a quick anti-inflammatory blast. These are now tools in your toolbox that you can use in any context, whenever you need them.

SHOULD YOU DO IT AGAIN?

Many of my clients become I-Burners again after they've been on a vacation where they ate a lot of food high in sodium and preservatives, or after airline flights that tend to make people swollen, or even after big temperature fluctuations in the weather. When it is hot and humid, the body has a hard time staying hydrated and may swell, holding on to water. When that happens, do the I-Burn plan again to get that excess water weight off quickly.

But even if you aren't travelling, doing the I-Burn periodically is so restorative and reparative that I recommend repeating it at least four times a year. Many of my clients do it at the beginning of every season, to reset their body in preparation for new foods and changing weather. If that's too often for you, I recommend it at the beginning of winter, a time when, according to Chinese medicine, the kidneys tend to be vulnerable to stress. Doing the I-Burn periodically is preventive. Or, do it therapeutically, whenever you notice the symptoms arising again. Your body will tell you when you need it.

CHAPTER SIX

D-Burn: Digestive Intervention

It's time to get your mucosal lining in tip-top shape. We'll be streamlining your digestion, clearing out your lungs and sinuses, and flooding you with energy. Get ready to banish the bloat, flaunt a flat belly and feel fantastic! You're my D-Burner now. Get ready to rock it.

READY . . .

If you know what's coming, you will be more likely to stay the course. Here is what will happen over the next five days:

- You will eat breakfast within thirty minutes of waking every day. This is crucial for the D-Burn because when you sleep, your respiration rate is low, your breathing is shallower and your bowels don't move (at least, they shouldn't!). When you get up and become more active, however, your breathing deepens and quickens and your body prepares to release waste that it's been holding all night long. By adding micronutrients to boost and fortify digestion and help maximize oxygen delivery even before things really get going, you will create a better environment for digestion and assimilation. This sets you up to digest your food and breathe better for the rest of the day.

- You will have one D-Burn Smoothie every day for breakfast, for a total of five D-Burn Smoothies over the course of the five days. Make your D-Burn Smoothie fresh each morning.

- You will have at least three cups of D-Burn Tea every day, for a total of at least fifteen cups over the course of the five days. You may brew this ahead of time in one big batch. Just warm up the tea as you need it.

- You will have two servings of D-Burn Soup each day (1 serving is 450g), for a total of 10 portions. The first serving will be your mid-morning snack. The second serving will be your mid-afternoon snack. This digestive-soothing soup will keep you from getting hungry between meals. You can also eat more of it, if 1 serving doesn't satisfy you. (In general, I tell my clients not to consume over 4 servings of soup per day. There is really no good reason to eat any more than that.) For this reason, your recipe will allow for some leftovers.

- You will have lunch and dinner each day, for a total of five lunches and five dinners. Each will consist of a cup of D-Burn Tea and a recipe from the D-Burn section in Chapter 9, or a serving each of vegetable, grain (115g) and protein from the D-Burn food list. If there are any foods on this plan that you can't eat or don't like, you can substitute any other foods from the same category on the food list at the end of this chapter. I suggest recipes for you to make and list them on the meal map and in the day-by-day descriptions, but the actual recipes are in Chapter 9. All lunch recipes serve one person, and all dinner recipes serve two people, unless I specify that you will be making more and saving some for a future meal. When this happens, I'll let you know when to stash half in the freezer and when to pull it out the night before you will need it so it can defrost. Of course, you can always double or triple any recipe if you also want to feed a *Burn* buddy or other family members with these delicious recipes.

- About one hour before bed each night, you will have a snack of cooked fruit. You know what they say about prunes and constipation? That applies to many types of cooked fruits. When you eat cooked fruits in the evening, this not only helps your bowels move the next morning, but it also soothes your gastrointestinal tract and feeds the good gut flora. This is a potent digestive remedy that will have a feel-good detoxifying effect.

· Note the free food list. You can add any of these foods to any meals or snacks at any time, if you need more food. The free D-Burn foods are:

- · D-Burn Soup
- · D-Burn Tea
- · Carrots
- · Cultured/fermented cabbage (purchased or homemade)
- · Cultured/fermented salsa (purchased or homemade)
- · Kale
- · Kimchi
- · Lemons
- · Limes

· Chew every bite of food at least fifteen to twenty times. This makes it easier on your digestive system, which is extra important on the D-Burn.

· You will drink half your body weight in ounces of water every day. I'll remind you throughout the day on your meal map and day-by-day schedule, but try to finish 25 per cent of your water by mid-morning, 50 per cent by lunch, 75 per cent by dinner and 100 per cent by bedtime. I prefer that you use high-quality spring water if you can. If this isn't possible, at least use some sort of purification system rather than plain tap water.

· Your day-by-day plan will include a daily Success Booster. You get to choose which ones fit best into your schedule and your life from the list of choices at the end of this chapter. (Find detailed descriptions of all Success Boosters with instructions for how to do them in Chapter 8.) These include specific D-Burn exercises; items to add to your smoothie, tea, or soup; and other easy as well as intense practices that will facilitate the work we are doing to your digestive and respiratory systems during the next five days.

· You will buy everything you need before you start so you are never stuck without the foods on the plan. Prepare your tea and soup ahead of time and keep them in the refrigerator. You can also prepare any of the meals ahead of time if you know you will be pressed for time and won't want to cook. I suggest you make your D-Burn Smoothie fresh every morning, for best flavour and nutrient punch.

- This chapter contains a grocery list for everything you will be eating on this plan. Remember that you can always substitute any food you don't like or can't have with any other food in the same category on the food list—a fruit for a fruit, a protein for a protein. Don't forget to add anything you will need for your chosen Success Boosters to your grocery list.

D-BURN GROCERY LIST

Be sure to check what you already have on hand before buying everything on this list. You probably already have some of these things in your freezer and pantry. Note that in some cases, we tell you a specific amount of something, such as 5 teaspoons chia seeds. We don't know in what size packages chia seeds (for example) might be available in your area, so we give you the specific amount you will need so you can buy the product in an appropriate size or determine whether you already have enough at home. Also, note that many health food stores

---

PORTION GUIDELINES

A special note about portion sizes: the portions for the recipes and the foods on the food lists are for anyone, man or woman, no matter how much weight you need to lose. All protein serving sizes are 110g for meat or poultry and 175g for seafood or fish. Do you need more if you are a man, or if you have more weight to lose? Actually, no. You only need enough protein to provide the building blocks for repair, and this amount is perfectly sufficient. If you feel like you need more food, remember that you can always have unlimited soup, tea and free foods. Fill up on soup and tea because they are powerful sources of repair. Water is filling, too, and you'll be drinking it a lot.

---

allow you to buy dry ingredients in bulk, so you can buy exactly the amount you need, if you have that option available to you.

Another reminder: if there is any food you don't like or cannot eat, that is not available in your area or not in season and just doesn't look very good, substitute it for any other food within the same category from the food list at the end of this chapter: fruit for fruit, vegetable for vegetable, protein for protein.

Free Foods

- D-Burn Soup
- D-Burn Tea
- Carrots
- Cultured/fermented cabbage (purchased or homemade— see page 185 for simple instructions on how to ferment your own veggies)
- Cultured/fermented salsa (purchased or homemade)
- Kale
- Kimchi
- Lemons
- Limes

Vegetables

- 700g asparagus
- 1 green bell pepper
- 3 red bell peppers
- 2 heads broccoli or 1 275g bag florets
- ½ head red cabbage
- 5 large carrots
- 1 head cauliflower
- 1 head celery
- 3 cucumbers
- 2 medium fennel bulbs
- 2 heads garlic
- 450g green beans
- 4 large spring onions
- 1 or 2 jalapeño peppers (more if you like your soup on the spicier side)
- 2 400g tins organic tomatoes, diced or whole
- 1 red onion
- 4 white onions
- 225g shiitake mushrooms
- 4 medium sweet potatoes
- 225g cherry tomatoes
- 2 yellow squash
- 6 medium courgettes (about 23cm long)

Fruit

- 3 green apples
- 6 lemons
- 1 lime
- 1 pear
- 150g prunes

Protein

- 450g lean minced beef
- 1 425g tin black beans
- 5 teaspoons chia seeds
- 175g flaxseeds
- 175g dried lentils
- 75g pine nuts
- 200g raw pumpkin seeds
- 50g dry quinoa
- 2 175g salmon fillets
- 2 tablespoons sesame seeds
- 450g sirloin or strip steak
- 450g minced turkey

Fats

- 3 tablespoons coconut oil
- 8 tablespoons grapeseed oil
- 9 tablespoons extra-virgin olive oil

Herbs, spices, sweeteners and miscellaneous

- 60g fresh basil
- 1 dried bay leaf
- 1 box beef or chicken broth
- ½ teaspoon black peppercorns
- 330ml chicken broth
- 1½ tablespoons chilli powder
- 1 teaspoon ground chipotle pepper
- 2 bunches fresh coriander or parsley, or enough to make 25g chopped
- 10 cinnamon sticks or 15 tablespoons ground cinnamon
- 4½ tablespoons coconut aminos or tamari (or any other gluten-free soy sauce)
- 2¼ teaspoons crushed red pepper flakes
- 3½ teaspoons ground cumin
- 1 12.5cm piece fresh ginger
- 10 bags licorice tea
- 1 bunch fresh mint
- ¼ teaspoon ground nutmeg
- 2½ teaspoons dried oregano
- ½ tablespoon paprika
- 1 bunch fresh parsley
- 10 bags peppermint or spearmint tea
- 1½ teaspoons dried rosemary
- 1½ tablespoons fresh rosemary
- 2 tablespoons tamari
- ¼ teaspoon dried thyme
- 3 tablespoons sea salt
- 1 900g carton vegetable or chicken broth (organic, non-dairy)
- Optional: birch xylitol or pure stevia

SET . . .

Are you ready to get cooking? It's very important to prep as much as you possibly can on the D-Burn plan. I often put my working-world clients on this plan. They don't have time for meal prep during the week because they are always at the office (even if it's a home office!). The more you make ahead of time, the smoother your week will go. Preparation will allow you to do the plan on autopilot while you focus on your career, family and life. Start on a Monday and by Friday, you won't believe how different you look and feel—and you will barely notice you were doing a plan!

It is important to make your D-Burn Tea and D-Burn Soup at least one day before you start, because this can take some time and you don't want to wake up and decide you don't have time to make the tea or make the soup for a snack. These, along with your D-Burn Smoothie, are the core of your food for the week. Portion them out into individual containers. Every morning, make your smoothie, warm up your tea and enjoy. If you work outside the home, bring a thermos of soup and one of tea to work with you, along with your lunch, which is usually leftovers from dinner the night before. All the recipes for your meals are in Chapter 9, so browse that section to see what you might want to make ahead of time.

This is also the time to choose your D-Burn Success Boosters. Find detailed descriptions of how to do these and what you will need in Chapter 8, but this list should allow you to choose what interests you so you can get everything you need.

D-BURN SUCCESS BOOSTERS

Exercise:
30 to 45 minutes of vigorous cardio, such as running, racquetball, aerobics class or spinning class

To Add to Your Smoothie:
70ml aloe vera juice

To Add to Your Tea:
1 pau d'arco tea bag

To Add to Your Soup:
150g chopped fennel

Easy Boosts:
Raw apple cider vinegar

Black walnut powder

Cultured/fermented vegetables

Detox bath with pau d'arco tea

Essential oil self-massage: oregano, nutmeg, peppermint, cardamom, clove

Flower essences

Neem oil

Oil pulling

Olive leaf extract

Reflexology

Soaking nuts, seeds, grains and legumes

Targeted D-Burn supplement protocol

Intense Boosts:
Dry sauna

Hot stone massage

Wheatgrass shots

Choose which five (or more) interest you, then check out Chapter 8 to see what you will be doing, exactly. You can do the same one every day, or pick five or more completely different Success Boosters, to keep it interesting. Make a place for these in your next five days, so you are sure to get one in every day. I'll make suggestions in your day-by-day about what you might want to try and when, but your Success Booster schedule is ultimately up to you.

GO!

Here are your D-Burn days, laid out step by step, by day and by meal. Everything should be in place now, and you should have all your supplies and all your foods. Remember that there are always negotiable items on *The Burn*. You can substitute foods you don't like, serving for serving, with foods you like within any given category (such as vegetable, fruit, or protein), but the smoothie, tea and soup are *required* for success on this plan. So are a minimum of one daily D-Burn Success Booster, for a total of at least five. Follow the plan, but make it yours. Let's get burning.

D-BURN PLAN, DAY-BY-DAY

YOUR D-BURN TO-DO LIST

☐ Did I get all the necessary ingredients for the recipes I will make?

☐ Did I prepare 15 cups (or more) of D-Burn Tea to keep in the refrigerator?

☐ Did I prepare 10 servings (or more) of D-Burn Soup to keep in my refrigerator?

☐ If I'm using bottled water, do I have enough to drink half my body weight in ounces each day for the next five days?

☐ Do I have everything I need to do my D-Burn Success Boosters?

D-Burn Daily Targets:
- Eat three meals and three snacks. Do not skip any of these, even if you aren't hungry.
- Drink half your body weight in ounces of water.
- Replace your regular cup of coffee or caffeinated tea with D-Burn Tea.
- If you get hungry between meals and snacks, or any meal or snack doesn't feel like enough, you can always have more D-Burn Soup, or any of the D-Burn-approved free foods (see the grocery list).
- Don't forget your daily D-Burn Success Booster.

D-BURN MEAL MAP

Here are your five days, at a glance. Snap a picture with your phone or make a copy and keep it with you so you always know what to eat.

DAY 1		
BREAKFAST		
SNACK		25%
LUNCH	Lentil Chilli (freeze half for Day 5 lunch)	50%
SNACK		75%
DINNER	Beef and Broccoli Bowl (save half for Day 2 lunch)	100%
SNACK	Stewed prunes (save half for Day 2 evening)	
AT A GLANCE	• 1 smoothie	
	• 3 cups tea	
	• 2 servings soup	
	• 1 cooked fruit	
	• Lentil Chilli	
	• Beef and Broccoli Bowl	
	• Half your body weight in ounces of water	
	• At least 1 Success Booster	

DAY 2

BREAKFAST

SNACK   25%

LUNCH Leftover Beef and Broccoli Bowl 50%

SNACK 75%

DINNER Shepherd's Pie (save half for Day 3 lunch) 100%

SNACK Leftover stewed prunes

AT A GLANCE
- 1 smoothie
- 3 cups tea
- 2 servings soup
- 1 cooked fruit
- Beef and Broccoli Bowl
- Shepherd's Pie
- Half your body weight in ounces of water
- At least 1 Success Booster

DAY 3

BREAKFAST

SNACK   25%

LUNCH   Leftover Shepherd's Pie   50%

SNACK   75%

DINNER   Stuffed Courgettes (save half   100%
for Day 4 lunch)

SNACK   Cooked pear (save half for Day 4 evening)

AT A GLANCE
- 1 smoothie
- 3 cups tea
- 2 servings soup
- 1 cooked fruit
- Shepherd's Pie
- Stuffed Courgettes
- Half your body weight in ounces of water
- At least 1 Success Booster

DAY 4

BREAKFAST

SNACK 25%

LUNCH Leftover Stuffed Courgettes 50%

SNACK 75%

DINNER Fennel and Salmon 100%

SNACK Leftover cooked pear
Defrost leftover Lentil Chilli from Day 1

AT A GLANCE
- 1 smoothie
- 3 cups tea
- 2 servings soup
- 1 cooked fruit
- Stuffed Courgettes
- Fennel and Salmon
- Half your body weight in ounces of water
- At least 1 Success Booster

DAY 5

BREAKFAST

SNACK 25%

LUNCH Leftover Lentil Chilli
(from Day 1 lunch) 50%

SNACK 75%

DINNER Italian Wonder 100%

SNACK ½ green apple, baked

AT A GLANCE
- 1 smoothie
- 3 cups tea
- 2 servings soup
- 1 cooked fruit
- Lentil Chilli
- Italian Wonder
- Half your body weight in ounces of water
- At least 1 Success Booster

DAY 1

When You Wake Up:
- Weigh yourself. You won't be doing this again until after the plan is over. Use this number to calculate how much water you will drink every day for the next five days: half your body weight in ounces. If you don't have a scale, just go by what you weighed at your last doctor's appointment.
- Schedule your Success Booster for the day. Maybe you'll kick off the D-Burn with a morning session of vigorous cardio, such as a spinning class or a jog through the park.

Breakfast:
1 serving **D-Burn Smoothie**
1 cup **D-Burn Tea**

Mid-morning Snack:
1 serving (450g) **D-Burn Soup**

Finish 25 per cent of your water.

D-Burn Nutrient Fact

Chia seeds come from a flowering plant in the mint family and are rich in alpha-linolenic acid. This fatty acid not only aids in healing the mucosal lining, but it also stimulates a specific metabolic pathway enhancing total body metabolism.

Lunch:
1 cup **D-Burn Tea**
1 serving **Lentil Chilli** (freeze half of the recipe for your Day 5 lunch)

If you do not want to make this recipe, or you prefer something else at lunch, you can also choose 1 portion each of vegetables, starch and protein from the food list at the end of this chapter, in addition to your D-Burn Tea.

Finish 50 per cent of your water.

Afternoon:

Finish 75 per cent of your water.

Afternoon Snack:

1 serving (450g) **D-Burn Soup**

Dinner:

1 cup **D-Burn Tea**
1 serving **Beef and Broccoli Bowl**

Set aside half the recipe for lunch tomorrow.

As with lunch, instead of this recipe, you may choose 1 portion each of vegetables, grain, and protein from the food list at the end of this chapter, in addition to your D-Burn Tea.

Evening Snack:

Combine 150g prunes, 110ml water, and a tablespoon of lemon juice. Simmer for 20 to 30 minutes, or until soft. Set aside half for tomorrow evening, and enjoy the rest about one hour before bedtime.

Evening:

Finish the rest of your water, if you haven't already.

Bedtime:

You might need to get up during the night to use the bathroom as your body adjusts to increased fluid intake, but be sure to get at least eight hours of sleep. This is crucial for digestive repair because digestion and peristalsis (the movement of your intestines to push food through) are regulated by the sympathetic nervous system. If you don't get deep sleep to support the parasympathetic nervous system, then the sympathetic nervous system won't be as efficient. So turn off the TV and hit the hay!

DAY 2

When You Wake Up:
- Measure out your water for the day—half your body weight in ounces. If you're having trouble remembering your water, put reminders in your phone throughout the day to keep you on track. Schedule your Success Booster for the day. How about trying oil pulling this morning before you brush your teeth?

Breakfast:
1 serving **D-Burn Smoothie**
1 cup **D-Burn Tea**

D-Burn Nutrient Fact
Ginger stimulates the release of digestive enzymes that help break down the nutrients in food. It also settles the stomach and gets rid of belly bloat.

Mid-morning Snack:
1 serving (450g) **D-Burn Soup**

Finish 25 per cent of your water.

Lunch:
1 cup **D-Burn Tea**
1 serving leftover **Beef and Broccoli Bowl**

Finish 50 per cent of your water.

Afternoon:
Finish 75 per cent of your water.

Afternoon Snack:
1 serving (450g) **D-Burn Soup**

Dinner:

1 cup **D-Burn Tea**

1 serving **Shepherd's Pie**

Set aside half the recipe for lunch tomorrow.

D-Burn Tip

Don't forget to chew your food fifteen to twenty times per bite! This is very important to make digestion easier.

Evening Snack:

Leftover stewed prunes, gently reheated

Evening:

A few hours before bed, finish the rest of your water. Also evaluate how you are feeling. Are you noticing any digestive changes? How is your bloating? You may already notice a flatter tummy.

Bedtime:

This is no time to skimp on sleep. Your body is undergoing major digestion renovation, so get your eight hours. If you are waking up too often to use the bathroom, try finishing your water two or three hours before bedtime.

DAY 3

When You Wake Up:

- Measure out your water for the day. Instead of filling glasses of water throughout the day, it helps to see exactly how much you need to drink, so you can meet your percentages and finish it all by evening. Schedule your Success Booster for the day. Maybe you'll add aloe vera juice to your D-Burn Smoothie, or pau d'arco tea to your D-Burn Tea.

Breakfast:

As you enjoy your breakfast, take just a few quiet, peaceful moments to prepare yourself and sip your smoothie and tea.

1 serving **D-Burn Smoothie**
1 cup **D-Burn Tea**

Mid-morning Snack:

1 serving (450g) **D-Burn Soup**

Finish 25 per cent of your water.

D-Burn Nutrient Fact

Red cabbage is rich in phytonutrients called flavonoids. Anthocyanin, the flavonoid that causes red cabbage to be dark red, reduces swelling in the GI tract and prevents cholesterol from becoming oxidized (or turning into the dangerous form of cholesterol) in the bowels.

Lunch:

1 cup **D-Burn Tea**
1 serving leftover **Shepherd's Pie**

Finish 50 per cent of your water.

Afternoon:

Finish 75 per cent of your water.

Afternoon Snack:

1 serving (450g) **D-Burn Soup**

Dinner:

1 cup **D-Burn Tea**

1 serving **Stuffed Courgettes**

Set aside half the recipe for tomorrow's lunch.

Evening Snack:

Cut up a pear into chunks and sprinkle it with a dash of nutmeg. Heat in a saucepan over low heat with a tablespoon of water until warm. Enjoy half before bed and save the other half for tomorrow night.

Evening:

A few hours before bed, finish the rest of your water. Also, evaluate how you responded to the recipes today. Are you noticing a difference when you eat certain kinds of foods and leave other foods out? Are you enjoying a break from gluten and dairy, or do you miss it? Pay attention to how your body responds to everything you eat, so you know your own digestion better.

Bedtime:

Get to bed early to fuel fat burning and digestive repair. That stewed fruit in the evenings should also help get everything moving smoothly by morning.

DAY 4

When You Wake Up:

- Measure out your water for the day. Are you getting used to drinking this much water, or is it still a challenge? Keep going. Water is incredibly important to facilitate digestion.
- Schedule your Success Booster for the day. How about something a little more challenging, like a wheatgrass shot?

Breakfast:

1 serving **D-Burn Smoothie**

1 cup **D-Burn Tea**

Mid-morning Snack:

1 serving (450g) **D-Burn Soup**

Finish 25 per cent of your water.

Lunch:

1 cup **D-Burn Tea**

1 serving leftover **Stuffed Courgettes**

Finish 50 per cent of your water.

Afternoon:

Finish 75 per cent of your water.

D-Burn Nutrient Fact

Fennel has been used for centuries as a lung and large intestine tonic in indigenous cultures and in medical systems like Chinese medicine and Ayurveda. It is high in water-binding fibre and is also used as a purgative to move the bowels.

Afternoon Snack:

1 serving (450g) **D-Burn Soup**

Dinner:

1 cup **D-Burn Tea**

1 serving **Fennel and Salmon**

Evening Snack:

Eat the other half of the pear you cooked yesterday evening.

Evening:

A few hours before bed, finish the rest of your water. Take the left-over Lentil Chilli from your Day One lunch out of the freezer to defrost for tomorrow. Also spend a few minutes evaluating your progress. How is that thick yellow fat? Is that heavy layer shrinking? Are you seeing more muscle tone and better skin? Do your lungs feel clearer? Note the changes so you can appreciate the benefits of your hard work.

Bedtime:

One more day to go! You are doing a great job. Get to bed and have sweet dreams about how hot you're going to look by the end of tomorrow.

DAY 5

When You Wake Up:
- Keep drinking that water! This is a habit you can hold on to, even when you are done with the D-Burn plan. It will always benefit you to drink half your body weight in ounces of water, whether you are on any kind of diet plan or not.
- Schedule your Success Booster for the day. A relaxing dry sauna or hot stone massage would be a lovely way to finish off the D-Burn.

Breakfast:
1 serving **D-Burn Smoothie**
1 cup **D-Burn Tea**

Mid-morning Snack:
1 serving (450g) **D-Burn Soup**

Finish 25 per cent of your water.

Lunch:
1 cup **D-Burn Tea**
1 serving leftover **Lentil Chilli**

D-Burn Nutrient Fact
Lentils, those little high-fibre legumes, prevent sugars from rapidly flowing from the GI tract into the bloodstream after a meal. They also stimulate the hormones that make you feel full.

Finish 50 per cent of your water.

Afternoon:
Finish 75 per cent of your water.

Afternoon Snack:
1 serving (450g) **D-Burn Soup**

Dinner:

1 cup **D-Burn Tea**
1 serving **Italian Wonder**

Evening Snack:

Take the last half of the green apple left over after making your Day 5 smoothie. Sprinkle it with cinnamon, then put it into a baking dish, add a tablespoon of water, cover and bake at 205°C/400°F for 20 minutes. Enjoy this for your evening snack.

Evening:

A few hours before bed, finish the rest of your water. You are a good night's sleep away from the end of the D-Burn, so take a good hard look in the mirror. Do you look different? Do you feel different? Pay particular attention to your belly, waistline, rib cage and upper back. Can you tell you've trimmed fat in these areas? Also, evaluate your energy. If you feel more energetic than you did before, consider which D-Burn habits you might want to carry with you into the rest of your life. The soup? The tea? The morning smoothie? Any of those awesome Success Boosters? They are all yours forever.

Bedtime:

It's the end of the fifth day and you are looking fully fabulous. Do you notice you are sleeping better now than you did at the beginning of the week? Get a good long sleep tonight and look forward to how great you'll feel and look in the morning.

D-BURN OPTIONS

As with all of these plans, I want you to follow what fits your preferences. You might not like or be able to eat every single food I've listed for you in the recipes for the D-Burn plan. That's OK. If you want to leave something out, you can substitute it with any item from the same category on the list. For example, if you hate asparagus, substitute cabbage, but not figs. You can have adzuki beans instead of buffalo, but not instead of bok choy.

This is your complete D-Burn food list. You know what I'm going to say next: if it's not on the list, then it is not a part of your next five days. Following this, find your list of all acceptable options for D-Burn Success Boosters.

D-Burn Food List

Free Foods

Eat as much as you want!

D-Burn Soup

D-Burn Tea

Carrots

Cultured/fermented cabbage
(purchased or homemade)

Cultured/fermented salsa
(purchased or homemade)

Kale

Kimchi

Lemons

Limes

Vegetables (minimum serving size is 150g raw)

Asparagus

Bell peppers (green and red)

Bok choy

Broccoli

Cabbage (green and red)

Carrots

Cauliflower

Celery

Chillies

Courgettes

Cucumber

Endive

Fennel

Garlic

Green beans

Jalapeño peppers

Leeks

Mushrooms (shiitake)

Onions, any type

Pumpkin

Shallots

Spinach

Spring greens

Spring onions

Squash, winter or summer	Turnips
Sweet potatoes	Watercress
Swiss chard	Yams
Tomatoes	

Fruits (serving size is 1 piece or 150g)

Fruits are for after dinner only and must be cooked, with the exception of the green apple in your smoothie, and lemons and limes for flavouring.

Asian pears	Papaya
Figs, fresh	Pears
Green apples	Pineapple
Lemons	Prunes
Limes	

Proteins (serving size is 110g meat or poultry; 175g fish; 1 egg; 75g beans; or 50g nuts or seeds)

Adzuki beans	Lamb
Almonds, raw	Lentils
Beef	Lima beans
Black beans	Pecans, raw
Brazil nuts, raw	Pine nuts, raw
Buffalo	Pistachios, raw
Cashews, raw	Pumpkin seeds, raw
Chia seeds	Salmon
Chicken	Sesame seeds, raw
Chickpeas	Sunflower seeds, raw
Eggs	Turkey
Elk	Walnuts, raw
Flaxseeds	Wild game (any kind)
Kidney beans	

Fats (serving size is 1 to 2 tablespoons)

Coconut oil	Extra-virgin olive oil
Grapeseed oil	

Grains (optional: serving size is up to 225g cooked)

Quinoa, sprouted	Wild rice, sprouted

Soaking and Sprouting

Some people have a hard time digesting grains because grains contain certain protective elements that hinder digestion. Soaking grains begins the sprouting process, which increases the cellulose and fibre content and makes the grain come alive by activating enzymes that were dormant. It's like adding water to a seed. It transforms the grain into a live plant. This washes away the hindering elements and activates those digestion-enhancing enzymes. I always recommend that grains be sprouted if possible, but this is important on the D-Burn, as we are repairing digestion. You can buy many grains already sprouted (the package will say if they are), or you can do it yourself. Just soak them in clean water in a glass jar at room temperature for twenty-four hours, then rinse and cook. This also works for seeds, nuts and legumes. Whatever you can sprout, go for it. Your digestion will thank you!

Miscellaneous (You may use fresh or dried)

Basil	Cumin
Bay leaf	Ginger
Birch xylitol	Kefir, non-dairy (purchased or
Black pepper	homemade)
Broth (beef, chicken, vegetable)	Kombucha (a kind of fermented
Chilli powder	tea)
Chipotle pepper	Licorice tea
Cinnamon	Mint
Clove	Nutmeg
Coriander	Oregano

What Is Kefir?

Kefir is similar to a thin drinkable yogurt and it contains healthful bacteria that your digestive tract will love. Look for unsweetened non-dairy types like coconut kefir, or make your own. Just purchase kefir grains, add them to coconut or almond milk and let the mixture sit at room temperature for 18 to 24 hours or in the refrigerator for one week. Strain out the grains and refrigerate the kefir. Drink it within five days. Many good websites will go into even more detail to tell you how to do this if you want to DIY.

Paprika

Parsley

Peppermint tea

Psyllium seed (gluten-free only)

Red pepper flakes, crushed

Rosemary

Sea salt

Stevia, pure

Tamari or coconut aminos

Thyme

Turmeric

YOU DID IT! NOW WHAT?

Congratulations! After five simple but intense days, you are feeling so much easier in your body. Your stomach will be flatter, your skin will look better, and you'll have a new level of energy. Your digestive system should be working better than before, too—your bowels moving more efficiently (ideally after every main meal). And those pesky five pounds you were lugging around last week? Sayonara, baby! Just look in the mirror—you look amazing! Now you are ready to go back to your regular routine, but keep any good habits and favourite recipes, to use whenever you need them. Getting through these last five days has been a real accomplishment, and you've learned a lot that you can continue to use in the future.

Many of my clients keep the D-Burn Smoothie, D-Burn Tea and D-Burn Soup in their back pockets to use even when they aren't doing *The Burn*. We all have those times when our digestive system gets a little backed up and we need some help. These are your new remedies, along with all the Success Boosters you've now got as notches on your proverbial belt. Break them out whenever you need them. I like to make a big batch of D-Burn Soup and keep it in the freezer for a quick and soothing meal. Portion it out and you can always bring it to work to tide you over, because you should be able to feel good in your belly *all* the time.

SHOULD YOU DO IT AGAIN?

If you ever feel any of your old symptoms creeping back in, or you want to go deeper into liquefying that stubborn yellow fat, just do the D-Burn again. It's the perfect antidote to an overindulgent weekend, when you get the sniffles, or as the perfect precursor to an event where belly-clinging clothes (or swimsuits!) are the order of the day. Many of my clients repeat the D-Burn plan on a schedule, such as once every season, or they break it out before or after vacations. Never forget how you felt before you did the D-Burn, and how you feel now. The D-Burn is always there for you.

H-Burn: Hormonal Intervention

It's time for a transformation! On the H-Burn plan, you will zero in on stubborn white fat as you target your liver, gallbladder and thyroid to normalize hormone function and rev up fat metabolism. But first, let's get all our ducks in a row.

READY . . .

First things first: knowing what's coming is crucial before you embark on your H-Burn journey. This is what's going to happen over the next ten days:

- You will eat breakfast within thirty minutes of waking every day, and as much as possible, at the same time every day. This is a critical practice on the H-Burn because hormones are all about rhythm and balance. We all have circadian rhythms that direct our bodies' processes through their natural fluctuations during a twenty-four-hour period, as well as over a 7-day and a 28-day period. When hormones are out of balance, this rhythm can also get out of sync. One way to help correct this is to establish a healthy and regular sleep-wake cycle. The sooner you infuse your body with micronutrients for encouraging hormone production and biosynthesis, the more your body will get the message that the sleep cycle is over and the waking cycle has begun. The H-Burn breakfast is a way to nurture your body and usher it into the day so the transition is a healthy one and sets the tone for a regular day of healthy rhythms. This in turn sets the tone for a regular and rhythmic week, which sets the tone for a regular and rhythmic month.

- You will have one H-Burn Smoothie every day for breakfast, for a total of ten H-Burn Smoothies over the course of the ten days. Make these fresh each morning. The recipe is in the H-Burn section of Chapter 9, as are all the recipes for the plan.

- You will have at least three cups of H-Burn Tea every day, for a total of at least thirty cups over the course of the ten days. You may brew this ahead of time in one big batch, but keep half in the freezer for the second half of the ten days so it stays fresh. The recipe in Chapter 9 is for fifteen cups and is meant to be made twice—once before you start, and once on Day 5.

- You will have two servings (1 serving is 450g) of H-Burn Soup each day for your morning and afternoon snacks, for a total of twenty servings. As with the tea, it's best to prep this ahead and store until ready to use. Freeze half, or make it in two batches. The good thing about this soup is that it is a concentrate, so it only makes half of what you need. Whenever you are ready to have soup, dilute 225g concentrate with 250ml water and reheat. This hormone-balancing soup will help you feel balanced and happy all day long. Eat more than two servings a day if you like what it does for you and/or you are still hungry. (As with the I-Burn, in general, I tell my clients not to consume over 4 servings of soup per day. There is really no good reason to eat any more than that.)

- You will eat a serving of fruit at lunch every day. I've made suggestions for you in the day-by-day list, but you can substitute any fruit you like from the H-Burn food list at the end of this chapter.

- You will have lunch and dinner each day, for a total of ten lunches and ten dinners. Each will consist of a cup of H-Burn Tea and a recipe from the H-Burn section in Chapter 9. Or, if you don't want to use the recipe, lunch is a serving each of vegetable, protein, fruit and fat from the H-Burn food list at the end of this chapter. Dinner is a serving each of vegetable, protein and fat from the H-Burn food list. Note that dinner does not contain fruit. If there are any foods on this plan that you can't eat or don't like, you can substitute any other foods from the same category on that list. You can also make any of these meals ahead of time. Just divide into single portions and freeze. All lunch recipes serve one person and all the dinner recipes serve two people, unless I ask you to make more because you will be setting aside and freezing half for a future meal. In these cases, I will let you know when to freeze and when to defrost. You can always double or triple any recipe to serve more people, if your family is joining in on the health benefits of *The Burn*. Just make allowances on your grocery list for any increase in amounts.

- If you are still hungry, you can always enjoy any of the free foods approved for the H-Burn plan. These are:

  - H-Burn Soup
  - H-Burn Tea
  - Celery
  - Cucumbers
  - Kale
  - Lemons
  - Limes
  - Mushrooms (all types)

- You will drink half your body weight in ounces of water every day. I'll remind you throughout the day on your meal map and day-by-day schedule, but try to finish 25 per cent of your water by mid-morning, 50 per cent by lunch, 75 per cent by dinner and 100 per cent by bedtime. I prefer that you use high-quality spring water if you can. If this isn't possible, at least use some sort of purification system rather than plain tap water.

- Your day-by-day plan will include ten Success Boosters over the ten days, but you may do as many as you like. These include customized exercise; items to add to your smoothie, tea or soup; and easy and also intense boosts that will facilitate the work we are doing to your hormonal system during the next ten days. You get to choose the ones you want to try, but each one is designed to encourage hormonal balance. Find a list in this chapter and a detailed description of how to do each one and what you need in Chapter 8.

- You will buy all the food and supplies you need ahead of time, based on the grocery list in this chapter, along with any substitutions you have decided on from the food lists at the back of this chapter, and anything you need for your Success Boosters.

Are you ready for your grocery list? Let's go to the store and load up the trolley. If this seems like too much, or to make sure your produce stays fresh, you can buy the food you need for the first half of the plan now, and then go shopping again in the middle of your ten days.

H-BURN GROCERY LIST

There are probably already many items on this list that you have, so don't be deterred by the length. Remember, this is ten days' worth, not just three or five. This list includes the exact amounts you will need for the ten days, so you can determine if you already have enough of something or how much you may need to buy. We won't try to guess what size packaging you have in your area, so go by what you will need, and use bulk bins to purchase exact amounts if your store has those.

Don't forget that you can always substitute any food you can't eat,

---

PORTION GUIDELINES

A special note about portion sizes: the portions for the recipes and the foods on the food lists are for anyone, man or woman, no matter how much weight you need to lose. Some people ask me about protein. All protein serving sizes are 110g for meat or poultry and 175g for seafood or fish. Do you need more if you are a man, or if you have more weight to lose? Actually, no. All you need is enough protein to provide the building blocks for repair, and this amount is perfectly sufficient. If you feel like you need more food, remember that you can always have unlimited soup, tea and free foods. Fill up on soup and tea in particular because they are powerful sources of repair. And don't forget your water!

---

can't find, or just don't like, with any other food in that same category—
vegetable for vegetable, fruit for fruit, fat for fat.

Free Foods

- H-Burn Soup
- H-Burn Tea
- Celery
- Cucumbers
- Kale
- Lemons
- Limes
- Mushrooms (all types)

Vegetables

- 1 tin artichoke hearts, in water
- 350g asparagus
- 450g beetroots
- 450g button mushrooms
- 2 heads cabbage
- 1 head cauliflower
- 2 heads celery
- 225g crimini mushrooms
- 3 medium fennel bulbs
- 4 heads garlic
- 1.25kg green beans
- 6 to 8 spring onions
- 1.50kg fresh kale
- 2 large leeks
- 1 package nori sheets
- 1 red onion
- 1 sweet onion (such as Vidalia)
- 5 yellow onions
- 1 head romaine lettuce
- 450g shiitake mushrooms
- 1 spaghetti squash
- 1.8kg fresh spinach
- 40g watercress
- 5 small yellow squash
- 12 courgettes

Fruit

- 10 whole grapefruit
- 3 lemons
- 15 limes
- 3 mangos
- 2 nectarines
- 3 oranges
- 2 peaches
- 4 plums
- 350g pomegranate seeds (2 to 3 pomegranates if you want to seed them yourself)

Protein

- 450g minced beef
- 350g skinless, boneless chicken breasts
- 2 bone-in, skin-on chicken thighs
- 2 cod fillets (175g each)
- 6 eggs
- 150g hummus
- 2 salmon fillets (175g each)

| 350g shrimp/prawns | 175g tinned tuna (in water) |

Fats

1 avocado	25g raw pine nuts
1 tin coconut milk	700g raw sunflower
1 jar coconut oil	seeds
8 kalamata olives	450g raw walnuts
12 tablespoons extra-virgin olive oil	

Herbs, spices, sweeteners and miscellaneous

3 teaspoons balsamic vinegar

1 bunch fresh basil

Black peppercorns

1 1-Litre carton chicken broth

1 bunch fresh coriander

14 bags dandelion root tea

1 bunch fresh dill

1 5cm piece fresh ginger

Horseradish

14 bags milk thistle tea

1 bunch fresh mint

1 tablespoon Dijon mustard

2 tablespoons grainy mustard

3 teaspoons dried oregano

2 bunches fresh curly parsley

1 tablespoon crushed red pepper flakes

1 bunch fresh rosemary

Sea salt

2 tablespoons plus 2 teaspoons tamari or coconut aminos

1 bunch fresh thyme

2 tablespoons turmeric

SET . . .

This is the longest plan, so your meal prep will involve larger amounts. You will make a *lot* of tea and soup for this plan, and you may not have a big enough pot or enough space in your refrigerator. I recommend either making the first half of your tea and soup before you start and the second half in the middle of your plan, or making it all at once but freezing half, so everything stays fresh. Make your smoothies fresh every morning. You might also want to make some or all of your lunches and dinners ahead of time, to make everything easier once you get started. Freeze everything in individual portions, label each one and then just pull out what you need the night before to defrost. Find all the recipes in the H-Burn section of Chapter 9. This is also the time to choose the ten (or more) Success Boosters for your H-Burn plan, so you know what you'll be doing and what you'll need. I've given you quite a range of choices, so pick those that seem appealing to you. Find detailed descriptions of everything you will do and everything you will need in Chapter 8. Remember, at least one per day, but you can always do more. These Success Boosters are powerful and will make a profound difference in your progress. Here are your H-Burn choices.

H-BURN SUCCESS BOOSTERS

If you don't like the Success Boosters I chose for you, or if you want to do more, then choose from this list.

Exercise:
H-Burn Exercise Bundle—three consecutive days of exercise rotating in a rhythm like this:

Day 1: Cardio
Day 2: Strength training
Day 3: Yoga or other stress-reducing activity

To Add to Your Smoothie:
1 raw organic egg (I especially like this for men struggling with testosterone levels. Buy organic and from a clean local source if you are worried about salmonella.)

To Add to Your Tea:
Essiac tea

To Add to Your Soup:
Yams

Easy Boosts:
Alternate nostril breathing
Black pepper
Dry skin brushing

Essential oil self-massage: sage, basil, ylang-ylang, geranium,
    frankincense
Flower essences
Chlorella
Hormone detox cocktail
Hydrotherapy (wet sock treatment)
Meditation
Milk thistle tincture
Pectin powder
Pomegranates and mulberries
Psyllium fibre
Reflexology
Sea vegetables and algae
Targeted H-Burn supplement protocol

Intense Boosts:
Castor oil packs
Clay bath
Infrared sauna
Ionic foot bath
Thai massage therapy

To find out all the details for how to do these and all other Success Boosters, check out Chapter 8. What appeals to you? What intrigues you? Why not give something a little bit daring a try? We're shaking things loose during the next ten days, and that can create some surprises in your body, so give yourself a boost!

GO!

Here you go. Everything is laid out for you step by step, day by day, meal by meal. All you have to do is follow the schedule. You have choices over the next ten days, but not about *everything*. You must have three meals and two snacks every day. No skipping! And you must have your smoothie, tea and soup. These are the core elements of your H-Burn plan, and they are absolutely required for stunning results.

H-BURN PLAN, DAY-BY-DAY

YOUR H-BURN TO-DO LIST

❏ Did I get all the necessary ingredients for the recipes I will make?

❏ Did I prepare my first 15 cups (or two 15-cup batches) of H-Burn Tea to keep in the refrigerator/freezer?

❏ Did I prepare 10 servings (or more) of H-Burn Soup concentrate, to keep in my refrigerator/freezer?

❏ If I'm using bottled water, do I have enough to drink half my body weight in ounces each day for the next ten days?

❏ Have I chosen and prepared for my ten or more H-Burn Success Boosters?

H-Burn Daily Targets:

· Eat three meals and two snacks. Do not skip any of these, even if you aren't hungry.

· Drink half your body weight in ounces of water.

· Replace your regular cup of coffee or caffeinated tea with H-Burn Tea.

· If you get hungry between meals and snacks, or any meal or snack doesn't feel like enough, you can always have more H-Burn Soup, H-Burn Tea or any of the H-Burn-approved free foods.

· Don't forget your daily H-Burn Success Booster.

H-BURN MEAL MAP

H-BURN

Here are your ten days, at a glance. Snap a picture with your phone or make a copy and keep it with you so you always know what to eat.

DAY 1

BREAKFAST

SNACK — 25%

LUNCH — Herbed Egg Salad, 1 peach — 50%

SNACK — 75%

DINNER — Pan-'fried' Chicken with Fennel and Walnuts (save half for Day 2 lunch) — 100%

AT A GLANCE
- 1 smoothie
- 3 cups tea
- 2 servings soup
- Herbed Egg Salad
- 1 peach
- Pan-'fried' Chicken with Fennel and Walnuts
- Half your body weight in ounces of water
- At least 1 Success Booster

H-BURN: HORMONAL INTERVENTION 129

DAY 2

BREAKFAST

SNACK 25%

LUNCH Leftover Pan-'fried' Chicken with Fennel and Walnuts 1 mango 50%

SNACK 75%

DINNER Coriander Shrimp/Prawns and Green Beans (freeze half for Day 5 dinner) 100%

AT A GLANCE
- 1 smoothie
- 3 cups tea
- 2 servings soup
- Pan-'fried' Chicken with Fennel and Walnuts
- 1 mango
- Coriander Shrimp/Prawns and Green Beans
- Half your body weight in ounces
- At least 1 Success Booster

DAY 3

BREAKFAST

SNACK   25%

LUNCH Chicken Avocado Salad with Creamy Coconut-Mango Dressing
2 plums 50%

SNACK 75%

DINNER Roasted Spaghetti Squash with Shiitake Mushrooms (save half for Day 4 lunch) 100%

AT A GLANCE
- 1 smoothie
- 3 cups tea
- 2 servings soup
- Chicken Avocado Salad with Creamy Coconut-Mango Dressing
- 2 plums
- Roasted Spaghetti Squash with Shiitake Mushrooms
- Half your body weight in ounces of water
- At least 1 Success Booster

DAY 4

BREAKFAST

SNACK 25%

LUNCH Leftover Roasted Spaghetti Squash with Shiitake Mushrooms 1 grapefruit   50%

SNACK 75%

DINNER Roasted Cauliflower and Salmon Defrost Coriander Shrimp/Prawns and Green Beans from Day 2 for tomorrow's dinner   100%

AT A GLANCE
- 1 smoothie
- 3 cups tea
- 2 servings soup
- Roasted Spaghetti Squash with Shiitake Mushrooms
- 1 grapefruit
- Roasted Cauliflower and Salmon
- Half your body weight in ounces of water
- At least 1 Success Booster

DAY 5

BREAKFAST

SNACK 25%

LUNCH Leftover Roasted Cauliflower and Salmon
1 nectarine
50%

SNACK 75%

DINNER Leftover Coriander Shrimp/ Prawns and Green Beans
100%

AT A GLANCE
- 1 smoothie
- 3 cups tea
- 2 servings soup
- Roasted Cauliflower and Salmon
- 1 nectarine
- Coriander Shrimp/Prawns and Green Beans
- Half your body weight in ounces of water
- At least 1 Success Booster

DAY 6

BREAKFAST

SNACK 25%

LUNCH Tuna Romaine Salad
1 peach   50%

SNACK 75%

DINNER Stuffed Cabbage Rolls with
Wild Mushroom Sauce
(save half for Day 7 lunch) 100%

AT A GLANCE
- 1 smoothie
- 3 cups tea
- 2 servings soup
- Tuna Romaine Salad
- 1 peach
- Stuffed Cabbage Rolls with Wild Mushroom Sauce
- Half your body weight in ounces of water
- At least 1 Success Booster

DAY 7

BREAKFAST

SNACK 25%

LUNCH Leftover Stuffed Cabbage Rolls with Wild Mushroom Sauce
1 mango 50%

SNACK 75%

DINNER Rosemary Chicken with Roasted Veggies
(freeze half for Day 10 dinner) 100%

AT A GLANCE
- 1 smoothie
- 3 cups tea
- 2 servings soup
- Stuffed Cabbage Rolls with Wild Mushroom Sauce
- 1 mango
- Rosemary Chicken with Roasted Veggies
- Half your body weight in ounces of water
- At least 1 Success Booster

DAY 8

BREAKFAST

SNACK 25%

LUNCH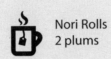

Nori Rolls
2 plums

50%

SNACK 75%

DINNER

Veggie Quiche
(save half for Day 9 lunch)

100%

AT A GLANCE
- 1 smoothie
- 3 cups tea
- 2 servings soup
- Nori Rolls
- 2 plums
- Veggie Quiche
- Half your body weight in ounces of water
- At least 1 Success Booster

DAY 9

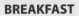

BREAKFAST

SNACK 25%

LUNCH Leftover Veggie Quiche
1 grapefruit
50%

SNACK 75%

DINNER Greek-Style Baked Cod
with Artichokes
Defrost the Rosemary Chicken
with Roasted Veggies from Day 7
dinner for tomorrow's dinner
100%

AT A GLANCE
- 1 smoothie
- 3 cups tea
- 2 servings soup
- Veggie Quiche
- 1 grapefruit
- Greek-Style Baked Cod with Artichokes
- Half your body weight in ounces of water
- At least 1 Success Booster

DAY 10

BREAKFAST

SNACK 25%

LUNCH Savoy, Watercress and Pomegranate Salad
1 nectarine
 50%

SNACK 75%

DINNER Leftover Rosemary Chicken
with Roasted Veggies
 100%

AT A GLANCE
- 1 smoothie
- 3 cups tea
- 2 servings soup
- Savoy, Watercress and Pomegranate Salad
- 1 nectarine
- Rosemary Chicken with Roasted Veggies
- Half your body weight in ounces of water
- At least 1 Success Booster

DAY 1

When You Wake Up:

- Weigh yourself today, but don't do it again until you are finished with this plan. I don't want you to focus on this number, which can fluctuate, especially as your hormones are beginning to understand that you are doing something different. Use this number as your starting point, and to calculate how much water you will drink every day for the next ten days: half your body weight in ounces. If you don't have a scale, just estimate your weight based on your last doctor's visit.

- Schedule your Success Booster for the day. I'd love it if you kicked off the H-Burn by launching into the Exercise Bundle. If you choose this particular Success Booster, that means 30 minutes of any cardio you enjoy today, 20 minutes of strength training tomorrow, and 30 to 60 minutes of yoga or other stress reducing exercise on Day 3.

Breakfast:

1 serving **H-Burn Smoothie**

1 cup **H-Burn Tea**

H-Burn Targeted Nutrition: Grapefruit

Rich in enzymes that burn fat and help intensify liver metabolism, grapefruit has a profound effect on the liver. However, make sure it is not contraindicated with any medication you might be taking, such as cholesterol medication.

Mid-morning Snack:

1 serving (450g) **H-Burn Soup**

Finish 25 per cent of your water.

Lunch:

1 cup **H-Burn Tea**

1 serving **Herbed Egg Salad**

1 peach

If you do not want to make this recipe, you can also choose 1 portion each of vegetables, protein, fruit and fat from the food list at the end of this chapter in addition to your H-Burn Tea.

Finish 50 per cent of your water.

Afternoon:

Finish 75 per cent of your water.

Afternoon Snack:

1 serving (450g) **H-Burn Soup**

Dinner:

1 cup **H-Burn Tea**

1 serving **Pan-'fried' Chicken with Fennel and Walnuts**

Have half of the recipe and save the other half for lunch tomorrow.

As with lunch, if you have already decided not to use a recipe, you may choose 1 portion each of vegetables, protein and fat from the food list at the end of this chapter, in addition to your H-Burn Tea.

Evening:

A few hours before bed, finish the rest of your water. Also notice how you are feeling. You've kicked off some interesting changes in your body, and you may already notice some. Be sure to notice mood changes as well as changes in your body composition over the next ten days.

For those of you who have trouble sleeping due to hormonal issues, losing sleep can be a vicious cycle that just makes hormonal issues worse. This is why hormonal repair is so crucial. If you are going to bed early enough but still having a problem getting to sleep or staying asleep, try adding an additional Success Booster to every day of your H-Burn plan and having an extra cup of H-Burn Tea before bed each

About Sleep on the H-Burn

Sleep is absolutely crucial for hormonal balance. Chronic sleep disruption or deprivation can imbalance your blood sugar levels and your endocrine function, and a study from the University of Chicago Medical Center concluded that sleep disruption can cause hormone levels to resemble those of someone of advanced age. Sleep deprivation stimulates the degradation of collagen and elastin, making skin sag and causing wrinkles. If you don't want to enjoy the effects of advanced ageing before you are of an advanced age, get at least eight hours of sleep per night. On the H-Burn, or for breaking through any really stubborn plateau, I would absolutely love it if you could get closer to ten hours.

night. You can also try the wet sock treatment form of hydrotherapy (see page 209).

Or try a supplement called DIM. Some people take supplements like melatonin or GABA to help them sleep, but I find that when sleep disturbance is hormonally based, DIM is more effective because it supports the pathways of hormone production, metabolism and biosynthesis. Instead of addressing sleep directly, it targets the mechanisms for sleep disturbance. Follow the dosage instructions on the particular formula you purchase.

DAY 2

When You Wake Up:
- Measure out your water for the day. Water is crucial for hormonal repair. All your systems need to be fully hydrated to work correctly, so drink up.
- Schedule your Success Booster for the day. If you are doing the Exercise Bundle, you will do 20 minutes of strength training today, but you could also choose to add some yummy yams to your H-Burn Soup.

Breakfast:
1 serving **H-Burn Smoothie**

1 cup **H-Burn Tea**

Mid-morning Snack:
1 serving (450g) **H-Burn Soup**

Finish 25 per cent of your water.

H-Burn Targeted Nutrition: Beetroots
Beetroots were used medicinally by the Romans as an aphrodisiac. They are high in a mineral called boron, which is directly related to the healthy production of sex hormones.

Lunch:
1 cup **H-Burn Tea**

1 serving leftover **Pan-'fried' Chicken with Fennel and Walnuts**

1 mango

Finish 50 per cent of your water.

Afternoon:
Finish 75 per cent of your water.

Afternoon Snack:

1 serving (450g) **H-Burn Soup**

Dinner:

1 cup **H-Burn Tea**
1 serving **Coriander Shrimp/Prawns and Green Beans**

Eat half the recipe and freeze the rest for your Day 5 dinner.

Evening:

A few hours before bed, finish the rest of your water. You've made it through two days—you might already be noticing an increased flushing of your system. You are probably using the bathroom more and you might notice that you have more energy. You might even feel warmer. That's a good sign that fat burning has commenced.

Bedtime:

Get to bed early to get your eight to ten hours. The more sleep you get on the H-Burn, the better. Sleep deprivation is a major cause of hormonal imbalance, so fix this one issue and you'll be helping your body achieve needed homeostasis.

DAY 3

When You Wake Up:

- Measure out your water for the day, and consider that all the excess hormones you've been producing because of hormone-induced weight gain can be flushed out of your body by sufficient water intake. Get those pesky waste hormones out!
- Schedule your Success Booster for the day. If you are doing the Exercise Bundle, it's yoga day, but wouldn't it also be nice to try some alternate nostril breathing? This is a practice that comes from yoga, so the two go perfectly together.

Breakfast:

1 serving **H-Burn Smoothie**

1 cup **H-Burn Tea**

H-Burn Targeted Nutrition: Milk Thistle and Dandelion Root Teas

Milk thistle and dandelion root are often paired because they are both such powerful liver tonics. Both have been used in folk medicine for centuries. Dandelion root is both a diuretic and a liver tonic that supports healthy liver function by maintaining hydration and electrolyte balance in the liver. Milk thistle contains flavolignans like silymarin that also maintain liver function and protect the liver from destruction by toxins and even poisons.

Mid-morning Snack:

1 serving (450g) **H-Burn Soup**

Finish 25 per cent of your water.

Lunch:

1 cup **H-Burn Tea**

1 serving **Chicken Avocado Salad with Creamy Coconut-Mango Dressing**

2 plums (note that plums are smaller than other fruits, so 2 plums equals 1
     fruit serving)

Finish 50 per cent of your water.

Afternoon:
Finish 75 per cent of your water.

Afternoon Snack:
1 serving (450g) **H-Burn Soup**

Dinner:
1 cup **H-Burn Tea**
1 serving **Roasted Spaghetti Squash with Shiitake Mushrooms**

Have half the recipe and save the rest for tomorrow's lunch.

Evening:
A few hours before bed, finish the rest of your water. Are you getting
used to all that water yet? Your body should eventually adjust so you
don't have to get up as often during the night. You might also be noticing a slimmer profile already, as water and your hormone-balancing
H-Burn meals emulsify that stubborn white fat.

Bedtime:
If you are having hormone-related sleep issues, make an effort to
create a routine around bedtime. This helps signal to your body that
it's time to wind down. Take a warm bath or shower, turn off electron-
ics such as the TV and computers, put away your phone and spend
the hour before bedtime doing something calm, such as meditating,
reading or relaxing with people you love. This kind of stress reduction
activity is enjoyable and amps up your success.

DAY 4

When You Wake Up:
- Keep drinking your water—it is helping with every single transformation process your body is trying to accomplish right now, especially detoxification, which is important as you liquefy fat cells and flush fat-soluble toxins out of your system. The cleaner your system is, the more easily it can repair all the mechanisms for hormonal production and biosynthesis.
- Schedule your Success Booster for the day. How about a Hormone Detox Cocktail this morning? That's an easy one, with a big impact.

Breakfast:
1 serving **H-Burn Smoothie**
1 cup **H-Burn Tea**

Mid-morning Snack:
1 serving (450g) **H-Burn Soup**

Finish 25 per cent of your water.

Lunch:
1 cup **H-Burn Tea**
1 serving leftover **Roasted Spaghetti Squash with Shiitake Mushrooms**
1 grapefruit

Finish 50 per cent of your water.

Afternoon:
Finish 75 per cent of your water.

Afternoon Snack:
1 serving (450g) **H-Burn Soup**

H-Burn Targeted Nutrition: Shiitake Mushrooms

Shiitake mushrooms and other wild mushrooms are common and potent remedies in Chinese medicine. Shiitake mushrooms in particular are a symbol of longevity, perhaps because they contain lentinan, which is an immune system strengthener used to fight disease, from the flu to cancer. Lentinan is also a liver protector, so it's great for the H-Burn, as it will help tonify your liver as you detox all those fat-soluble toxins you've been storing.

Dinner:

1 cup **H-Burn Tea**
1 serving **Roasted Cauliflower and Salmon**

Eat half and save the other half for lunch tomorrow.

Evening:

Sometime this evening, take the remaining Coriander Shrimp/Prawns and Green Beans out of the freezer so it can defrost for tomorrow's dinner. A few hours before bed, finish the rest of your water.

This is also a good time to evaluate your progress. As you detox, you may feel a few temporarily unpleasant symptoms, like stinky sweat and low energy, but these are all about to turn around, so don't let those deter you. The toxins are coming out, and you know what they say—better out than in!

Bedtime:

Several studies have linked accelerated ageing in the body with lack of sleep. Yikes! There is no reason to rush the clock or the calendar. Getting eight to ten hours of sleep can seem to *reverse* the clock, so hit the hay and wake up looking younger tomorrow.

DAY 5

When You Wake Up:
- Measure out your water for the day. Another important reason to drink lots of water on the H-Burn is to assist your liver, which is doing extra work right now, processing toxins you are banishing from your system. Extra water will ease the burden, diluting the toxins so they are easier to manage.
- Schedule your Success Booster for the day. Dry skin brushing before your shower is a quick and powerful way to boost your toxin removal.

Breakfast:
1 serving **H-Burn Smoothie**
1 cup **H-Burn Tea**

Mid-morning Snack:
1 serving (450g) **H-Burn Soup**

Finish 25 per cent of your water.

Lunch:
1 cup **H-Burn Tea**
1 serving leftover **Roasted Cauliflower and Salmon**
1 nectarine

Finish 50 per cent of your water.

Afternoon:
Finish 75 per cent of your water.

Afternoon Snack:
1 serving (450g) **H-Burn Soup**

Dinner:
1 cup **H-Burn Tea**
1 serving leftover **Coriander Shrimp/Prawns and Green Beans**

H-Burn Targeted Nutrition: Cauliflower

Cauliflower is a cruciferous vegetable with lots of vitamin C, vitamin K, folate and B vitamins, as well as fibre. It can help bind toxins as they are released and carry them out of the body. There is also some evidence that cauliflower can help the body fight hormone-related cancers. That's likely because of the broad range of antioxidants it contains, which can protect cells from the stress of oxidation as you are detoxing. The phytonutrients it contains, especially gluconasturtiin, activate detoxifying enzymes in the body.

Evening:

A few hours before bed, finish the rest of your water. And congratulate yourself! You've made it halfway through the ten days. Continue to notice how you feel as you eat the H-Burn foods. Are there any particular meals you love? Are you getting addicted to that H-Burn Smoothie? Is the soup your new favourite snack? How does your body respond when you eat the H-Burn foods, and also how is your body responding now that you *aren't* eating a lot of the metabolism killers you probably ate before, like wheat, soy, corn and sugar? Don't take good feelings for granted. Notice why you have them. These are messages from your body about what it likes.

Bedtime:

When you sleep, your body goes through major repair. It builds muscle and processes toxins from the day. If you don't give it enough time, you won't detox or build structure sufficiently. Eight hours, minimum. But see if you can sneak in another hour or two tonight.

DAY 6

When You Wake Up:

- By now you know the drill—don't forget your water! A squeeze of lemon can help your liver produce bile and trigger your morning bathroom time.
- Schedule your Success Booster for the day. Is it time to start another Exercise Bundle and kick off the second half of the ten days with another day of fun cardio, such as a bike ride or a kickboxing class?

Breakfast:

1 serving **H-Burn Smoothie**

1 cup **H-Burn Tea**

Mid-morning Snack:

1 serving (450g) **H-Burn Soup**

Finish 25 per cent of your water.

Lunch:

1 cup **H-Burn Tea**

1 serving **Tuna Romaine Salad**

1 peach

Finish 50 per cent of your water.

H-Burn Targeted Nutrition: Chickpeas

Chickpeas, also called garbanzo beans, have a high fibre content. This is important when your body is trying to eliminate a lot of fat-soluble toxins, since the fibre binds with the bad stuff and carries it out. Chickpeas are also stars at balancing blood sugar and insulin, which can help stabilize mood and energy. They also contain a particular combination of phytonutrients—flavonoids such as quercetin, kaempferol and myricetin, as well as phenolic acids and anthocyanins, which all contribute to a potent healing effect.

Afternoon:

Finish 75 per cent of your water.

Afternoon Snack:

1 serving (450g) **H-Burn Soup**

Dinner:

1 cup **H-Burn Tea**
1 serving **Stuffed Cabbage Rolls with Wild Mushroom Sauce**

Eat half the recipe and save the rest for lunch tomorrow.

Evening:

A few hours before bed, finish the rest of your water. Also, consider how your moods have changed. Are you feeling more patient, more even, calmer? Maybe you notice you are less irritable with family members or yourself, or your brain fog has cleared and you are thinking more sharply and clearly. These are all positive signs that you are detoxing and that your hormones are getting back into balance, so keep going!

Bedtime:

Sleep also impacts your mental health. Your brain rests, repairs and processes thoughts and feelings while dreaming. If you aren't getting enough sleep, you can feel more stressed, impatient, anxious, or frustrated. Let sleep work its magic on your mood.

DAY 7

When You Wake Up:
- Measure your water out for the day and shake things up a bit. Maybe throw an orange slice in there, or a handful of pomegranate seeds.
- Schedule your Success Booster for the day. Perhaps you'll try an essential oil self-massage, or a reflexology foot massage, using any of the H-Burn essential oils. If you are doing the Exercise Bundle, it's strength training day.

Breakfast:
1 serving **H-Burn Smoothie**
1 cup **H-Burn Tea**

Mid-morning Snack:
1 serving (450g) **H-Burn Soup**

Finish 25 per cent of your water.

Lunch:
1 cup **H-Burn Tea**
1 serving leftover **Stuffed Cabbage Rolls with Wild Mushroom Sauce**
1 mango

Finish 50 per cent of your water.

Afternoon:
Finish 75 per cent of your water.

Afternoon Snack:
1 serving (450g) **H-Burn Soup**

Dinner:
1 cup **H-Burn Tea**
1 serving **Rosemary Chicken with Roasted Veggies**

Enjoy half this recipe and freeze the other half for your Day 10 dinner.

Evening:

A few hours before bed, finish the rest of your water. Then look at your face. How does your neck look? Your skin should be tightening up and looking firmer and less saggy.

Bedtime:

How are you doing with your stress management efforts? Remember that you can always do multiple Success Boosters in one day. Maybe a relaxing evening with some visualization will set the stage for a good night's sleep. After you get into bed, settle down, close your eyes and imagine the most calming and relaxing environment you can, in as much detail as you can. This is a great way to drift off to sleep.

DAY 8

When You Wake Up:
- Measure out your water and imagine every sip is flushing out fat.
- Schedule your Success Booster for the day. Maybe this is a good day to try something a little more extreme, such as a castor oil pack or a clay bath. If you are doing the Exercise Bundle, it's also yoga day, which can calm you and prepare you for a more interesting Success Booster you haven't tried before.

Breakfast:
1 serving **H-Burn Smoothie**

1 cup **H-Burn Tea**

Mid-morning Snack:
1 serving (450g) **H-Burn Soup**

Finish 25 per cent of your water.

Lunch:
1 cup **H-Burn Tea**

1 serving **Nori Rolls**

2 plums

Finish 50 per cent of your water.

Afternoon:
Finish 75 per cent of your water.

Afternoon Snack:
1 serving (450g) **H-Burn Soup**

Dinner:
1 cup **H-Burn Tea**

1 serving **Veggie Quiche**

Eat half of this recipe and save the other half for tomorrow's lunch.

H-Burn Targeted Nutrition: Whole Eggs

Whole eggs, especially those that are pasture-raised (instead of from chickens confined to an enclosure), are rich sources of omega-3 fatty acids, vitamin E, choline and selenium, as well as high-quality protein you need to build muscle. Eggs are also a source of cholesterol, which sounds bad, but actually is not—your body needs cholesterol for healthy hormone production, so this is essential on the H-Burn for both men and women.

Evening:

A few hours before bed, finish the rest of your water. Also, do an overall evaluation. Is your hair shinier and less crispy? Is your skin looking more supple and less dry? Are your legs slimming down? How much weight have you lost? And are you feeling a resurgence of energy, good mood, even libido? These are all the wonderful gifts of the H-Burn. Pay attention to them, so you will appreciate them more.

Bedtime:

Your body *loves* sleep, and so do your hormones, so get to bed on time. If you've been sleeping more than usual, have you noticed that it has been worthwhile in terms of your energy, productivity and mood during the day? I hope you will make getting more sleep a higher priority in your life, even after the H-Burn.

DAY 9

When You Wake Up:
- The H-Burn plan may soon be coming to an end, but you don't need to end your water-drinking habit. Keep that up every day from now on! It's great for facilitating the work of your metabolism.
- Schedule your Success Booster for the day. What about something funky like the wet sock treatment? You'll be surprised how good you'll feel in the morning.

Breakfast:
1 serving **H-Burn Smoothie**
1 cup **H-Burn Tea**

Mid-morning Snack:
1 serving (450g) **H-Burn Soup**

Finish 25 per cent of your water.

Lunch:
1 cup **H-Burn Tea**
1 serving leftover **Veggie Quiche**
1 grapefruit

Finish 50 per cent of your water.

Afternoon:
Finish 75 per cent of your water.

Afternoon Snack:
1 serving (450g) **H-Burn Soup**

Dinner:
1 cup **H-Burn Tea**
1 serving **Greek-Style Baked Cod with Artichokes**

H-Burn Targeted Nutrition: Artichokes

Artichokes are another high-fibre vegetable and another plant that has been used medicinally for centuries. They are good at supporting the liver and gallbladder because they increase healthy bile flow and fat digestion. They contain the antioxidants cynarin and silymarin, both of which may protect and regenerate the liver when it is damaged.

Evening:

Take the Rosemary Chicken with Roasted Veggies left over from Day 7 out of the freezer so it can defrost for tomorrow's dinner. A few hours before bed, finish the rest of your water. Notice whether your sugar cravings have diminished. Sugar cravings are a common issue when hormones are out of balance, but if you notice you suddenly aren't quite so mad to get your sugar fix, that's a good sign that your hormones are getting back to where they should be.

Bedtime:

One more day to go! Make the most of it by trying to get nine or ten hours of sleep tonight. It will pay off tomorrow.

DAY 10

When You Wake Up:
- Measure out your water and finish every drop today. You can do it!
- Schedule your Success Booster for the day—and I hope it's not your last one! A Thai massage would be awesome, but if that's not in your stars, consider a relaxing ionic foot bath or an infrared sauna for maximum stress relief. Remember that you can continue to do any of the H-Burn Success Boosters, even when you aren't doing the plan.

Breakfast:
1 serving **H-Burn Smoothie**
1 cup **H-Burn Tea**

Mid-morning Snack:
1 serving (450g) **H-Burn Soup**

Finish 25 per cent of your water.

Lunch:
1 cup **H-Burn Tea**
Savoy, Watercress and Pomegranate Salad
1 nectarine

Finish 50 per cent of your water.

Afternoon:
Finish 75 per cent of your water.

Afternoon Snack:
1 serving (450g) **H-Burn Soup**

Dinner:
1 cup **H-Burn Tea**
1 serving leftover **Rosemary Chicken with Roasted Veggies**

Evening:

A few hours before bed, finish the rest of your water. You also might consider scheduling your annual checkup, to see if your cholesterol, triglycerides, blood sugar and blood pressure have gone down. If any of those numbers were high for you, I'd bet money they've gone down after ten days on the H-Burn.

Bedtime:

You are amazing! Ten full days, and you've shifted your shape, soothed your mood and restored your energy. Instead of partying all night to celebrate, get to bed early so you look completely ravishing in the morning. That will be the time to do another once-over in the mirror and pat yourself on the back for looking and, even more importantly, *feeling* so awesome.

H-BURN OPTIONS

You might not like or be able to eat every food I've listed for you in the recipes. If you want to leave something out, you can substitute with any item from the same food category list. Maybe you hate beetroots but you love artichokes or spinach. No problem! Here are all the foods you can eat during the next ten days. If it's not on the list, then it is not a part of your plan. After this is your list of all acceptable options for H-Burn Success Boosters.

H-Burn Food List

Free Foods

Eat as much as you want!

H-Burn Tea	Kale
H-Burn Soup	Lemons
Celery	Limes
Cucumbers	Mushrooms (all types)

Vegetables (minimum serving size is 150g raw)

Artichoke hearts (fresh or water-packed)	Leeks
Asparagus	Mushrooms (button, crimini, shiitake)
Beetroots	Onions (red, sweet, yellow)
Cabbage, red or green	Romaine lettuce
Cauliflower	Sea vegetables (dulse, kelp, kombu, nori)
Celery	
Courgettes	Spaghetti squash
Cucumbers	Spinach
Fennel	Spring onions
Garlic	Watercress
Green beans	Yellow squash
Kale	

Fruits (serving size is 1 piece or 150g)

Grapefruit	Nectarines
Lemons	Mangos
Limes	Mulberries

Oranges

Peaches

Plums (because they are smaller
than other orchard fruits,
serving is 2 plums)

Pomegranates

Proteins (serving size is 110g meat or poultry; 175g fish or seafood; 2 eggs; or 110g hummus)

Beef

Chicken

Cod

Eggs

Hummus

Mussels

Salmon

Shrimp/Prawns

Tuna

Fats (serving size is ¼ avocado; 1 to 2 tablespoons coconut milk or oil; 50g olives; 50g nuts or seeds)

Avocado

Coconut milk (canned)

Coconut oil

Olives

Extra-virgin olive oil

Pine nuts, raw

Sunflower seeds, raw

Walnuts, raw

Miscellaneous

Balsamic vinegar

Basil, fresh

Black pepper

Chicken broth

Coriander, fresh

Dandelion root

Dill, fresh

Ginger, fresh

Horseradish

Milk thistle

Mint, fresh

Mustard, Dijon and grainy

Oregano, dried

Parsley, fresh

Red pepper flakes, crushed

Rosemary, fresh

Sea salt

Tamari

Thyme, fresh or dried

Turmeric

YOU DID IT! NOW WHAT?

Congratulations! You may have experienced ups and downs, easy days and difficult days over the last week, but now you can see how much it has paid off in real results. Take a good hard look in the mirror. Try on some clothes that didn't fit right before. Your body has sculpted itself back into shape by trimming the hormone-induced fat in all the right places. I bet you look and feel absolutely fabulous, so go out and flaunt it, but keep any good habits and favourite recipes you've acquired over the past ten days, to use whenever you need them.

I'm proud of you as you finish the H-Burn because this is one of the most difficult plateaus to overcome. If the I-Burn means wading through water and the D-Burn is like wading through mud, the H-Burn is the equivalent to wading through cement. This is the hardest fat to lose, no contest, and the most stubborn weight loss resistance comes from hormonal imbalance.

If you've broken through your plateau and the scale is moving again, and if your moods feel more stable, then you've accomplished what we set out to accomplish with the H-Burn. We want to get you back in weight loss mode. Even if you haven't finished losing all the weight you need to lose, you can go back to your regular weight loss regimen or healthy eating and exercising lifestyle in a positive way. If you've ever had your car stuck in mud or snow, you know that sometimes it takes some boards or a bag of kitty litter and some people with strong backs to push it out. Once the car is unstuck, it doesn't mean you are at your destination yet, but it does mean that getting to your destination is now possible. You are back on track to long-term weight loss and hormonal balance. I consider any weight loss at all on the H-Burn to spell success because it means you are moving toward your goal again. Make the most of this victory and that down-shifting number. If you've become unstuck from hormonal weight loss resistance, you have done something *major*. This is huge.

If you are now at your ideal weight, or you never had that much weight to lose, then revel in all the other great things the H-Burn has done for your body—your hormones are settling back into balance because you've nourished and activated the systems that keep them in production and that use your hormones the way they are meant to be used. If healing is evident in your body after the H-Burn, that's a major success, because it means that now all levels of healing are possible. So a high five and a big shout-out to you! You've come through the worst of the worst plateaus, and you can feel great knowing that you've broken through. People spend thousands of dollars on diets and countless hours at the gym and if their hormonally based weight loss resistance isn't fixed, it will all be for nothing. If your hormones are out of whack, you're not going to have the success you deserve.

But you did it. *You* did it.

And you can keep doing it. Many of my clients keep the smoothie, tea and soup in their rotation, even when they aren't doing *The Burn*. Everyone gets hormonal once in a while. Our hormones rule us, and sometimes we make choices (or they get made for us thanks to PMS, adolescence, pregnancy, perimenopause and menopause) that throw us out of whack. A day or two of H-Burn Smoothies, Teas and/or Soups can help you feel like yourself again. Keep batches in the freezer for hormonal emergencies.

SHOULD YOU DO IT AGAIN?

Many of my clients repeat the H-Burn plan whenever they get PMS-y or notice any signs of hormonal weight gain. If you're going through menopause, you may want to come back to it every few months, just to keep yourself on track.

I like to use the H-Burn in this way for my menopausal clients to support and balance the body while it is going through this important transition. In Chinese medicine, menopause is a time when the creative energy being used in your body for fertility moves into your heart. Now it's time to start creating other beautiful things just for you. When you are finished with menopause, the body can rest in homeostasis, and it can be a beautiful transition if you give your body everything it needs to get through it.

CHAPTER EIGHT

More Kindling: Success Boosters

S uccess Boosters are close to my heart. Over the years, I have col-lected these holistic folk and home remedies, as well as other natural medicine strategies. I consider myself somewhat of a remedy collector. I am always willing to try something new, but I keep it in my collection only if it really works. I want tangible results. In this chapter are the remedies I have found that effect the most profound changes in my clients. They can help you, too.

Each of these remedies works best for a certain goal, which is why I have divided them into the I-Burn, D-Burn and H-Burn sections. Although many remedies have multiple benefits and could be useful for more than one of the plans, I have put them where I like to use them, according to the benefits I feel are most useful and active. You will also note that in a few cases, Success Boosters appear in more than one category. Often they are used differently in each category. For ex-ample, all the plans have an essential oil option and a Bach flower rem-edies option, but the oils and flower remedies I use for the I-Burn differ from those I like for the D-Burn and those that I feel work best for the H-Burn.

I have given you a variety of Success Boosters under each plan for good reason—there are many different options because I want you to choose what you are most comfortable with. Don't do something you don't want to do, but I encourage you to be curious and expand your horizons a bit. If something sounds intriguing, give it a try!

My only word of caution is this: if you have a serious medical condition, are on prescription medication, or are pregnant or nursing, check with your doctor about any specific remedies you want to try, to make sure it is OK for you and your situation.

Within each plan in this chapter, I have divided the Success Boosters into several categories:

- Targeted exercises.
- Additions to your smoothie.
- Additions to your tea.
- Additions to your soup.
- Easy boosts you can do on your own.
- Intense boosts that require special equipment or that may be a little more difficult or have a stronger, more potent effect. These are not for everyone, but they might be just right for you. Give them a read and see what you think.

Each Success Booster includes a description of what it is, what it does in your body, the tools or supplies you will need to do it and step-by-step instructions for how to do it. The Success Boosters for your plan will super-charge your weight loss and enhance the effects of the food on your plan. They truly are boosters for what we are trying to accomplish.

For each plan, choose one for each day, or more if you like. You could do the same one for all the days, or choose a different one every single day—you've got a Success Booster smorgasbord that you can carry with you after you're done with your *Burn* plan. They are all therapeutic and beneficial. If you love something you find here, keep it in your toolbox the way I do and keep calling on it whenever you need it. Let your favourites become a part of your life.

I know you will enjoy incorporating these into your plan and into your life, as much as my clients do.

I-BURN SUCCESS BOOSTERS

I-Burn Success Boosters are designed to do one or more of the following:

- Reduce your stress hormones
- Hydrate your body
- Scavenge subcutaneous fat or cellulite
- Encourage excretion through the lymphatic system
- Encourage excretion through the kidneys and bladder
- Help tip your body to a more alkaline state
- Deliver intensive micronutrients to the kidneys, lymphatic system and/or bladder

EXERCISE BOOST

On any day you choose to exercise, I prefer you do so before 2:00 p.m. for maximum benefit. The body has natural wake and rest cycles and you are most metabolically active before 2:00 p.m. After this time, your body begins to shift into more of a rest-and-repair mode. This is why many people feel their energy ebb in the afternoon. We want to take advantage of these natural rhythms in the body to maximize our workout efforts. Exercising after 2:00 p.m., however, is still better than not exercising at all. You will still receive many benefits from afternoon or even evening exercise. Don't exercise within an hour of your normal bedtime. It's counterproductive. Come bedtime, there is only one kind of cardio you should be doing . . . ahem. Otherwise, I don't want to hear about it. Bedtime is bedtime and exercise will be more of a stressor at this time.

Although no one Success Booster is required, I strongly encourage you to include exercise Success Boosters as part of your I-Burn experience, if you can. It really is a powerful adjunct to your body's efforts to fight reactivity, inflammation and fluid retention.

Walking

The goal of exercise on the I-Burn plan is to increase circulation in a relaxed, low-stress way, and no exercise does that better than walking. Walking will get fluid moving out of your body, will help ignite the burning of subcutaneous fat, and is also relaxing and pleasant. Walking outside is the best option. Sweating it out on a treadmill at the gym while staring at a television isn't what we're going for here. I want you breathing fresh air, looking at nature and moving your body in a natural, easy way that feels rejuvenating rather than exhausting.

What You Need:
- A supportive pair of exercise shoes
- An appropriate outdoor (preferably) or indoor (better than nothing) environment for walking

Step by Step:
Lace up your shoes, head outside and walk at a leisurely-to-brisk pace for 30 minutes.

Yoga

Stress leads to inflammation, and on the I-Burn we want to go in the opposite direction, easing the body into a supported and nurtured state to help cool inflammation and signal to the body that fat storage isn't necessary and fat burning is A-OK. Yoga is an ancient practice for yoking the mind and body together through meditation, and certain kinds of movements meant to help master the body grew out of this goal. Today we use those movements without necessarily thinking about the original purpose of yoga. Yet even when we don't think about it, yoga exercises (called *asanas*) align the body and calm the mind. Yoga has an anti-inflammatory as well as an anti-swelling effect. Not only are the exercises calming, but the poses elongate your muscles, strengthen and adjust joints, and compress and then release organs in a way that helps get lymph flowing more freely through the body. Whether you do yoga at home with a book or DVD or freestyle, or you take a yoga class, you will get great benefits.

What You Need:
- Loose-fitting clothes
- A yoga mat (also called a sticky mat)
- A yoga book, DVD or class

Step by Step:

It's best to learn yoga first from a qualified teacher who can make sure you are doing the movements correctly, so sign up for a class or get a good DVD. Ask your yoga-fan friends for recommendations. The following yoga poses are good for you on the I-Burn:

- Downward-facing dog
- Mountain pose
- Pigeon pose
- Shoulder stand (if you don't have any neck or back issues)
- Triangle pose
- All twisting poses (poses that rotate your torso)
- All inversions (poses that put your feet above your head). Some yoga teachers say you should not do inversions under certain conditions, like during your period or if you have certain injuries. Talk to your yoga instructor if you have any doubts about doing inversions. Listen to your body and your teacher.

I-BURN SMOOTHIE BOOST

Kale or Spinach

Kale and spinach are potent sources of nutrients. These leafy greens are rich in many vitamins, minerals and phytochemicals that reduce inflammation and encourage detoxification, such as vitamins C, A and E, and the B vitamins; calcium, potassium, magnesium; a wide variety of anti-inflammatory flavonoids and carotenoids; and omega-3 fatty acids. The isothiocyanates in kale have demonstrated cellular detoxification action. Pop them into your I-Burn Smoothie for an extra anti-inflammatory boost.

What You Need:
- 225g fresh kale leaves, spinach leaves, or baby spinach leaves

Step by Step:
1. Wash the greens. Tear kale leaves away from the thick stem, and throw away any long, tough spinach stems. Tear the larger leaves into pieces. (If using baby spinach, you don't have to do anything to the leaves except clean them.)
2. Add 225g greens to your regular I-Burn Smoothie, blend and drink.

DIY Dandelion Tea

If you have unsprayed dandelions in your garden, you can harvest the young greens before the plant flowers and make tea from the fresh or dried leaves (dry them on a tray in the sun, in an oven on low heat or in a dehydrator). Just put some leaves in a teapot, pour boiling water over them, let them steep for about 5 minutes, strain and drink.

I-BURN TEA BOOST

Dandelion Tea

This potent but pleasant tea is made from dandelion leaves (note: this is a different remedy from dandelion root tea, which is more of a liver tonic and is used on the H-Burn). I use dandelion tea for I-Burns because it is a potent diuretic that relieves swelling, oedema and water retention. It also nourishes you with vitamin C, vitamin A and potassium, as well as trace minerals.

What You Need:
- Loose dandelion tea or dandelion tea bag; you'll need 2 to 3 teaspoons or 1 tea bag per cup
- Tea ball or other device for preparing loose tea, if you aren't using a tea bag
- Boiling water or heated I-Burn Tea

Step by Step:

1. Use 2 to 3 teaspoons of dandelion leaf tea per cup of boiling water or I-Burn Tea.

2. Steep tea leaves for 3 to 5 minutes in your I-Burn Tea (or separately in hot water), then drink.

I-BURN SOUP BOOST

Beetroot Greens

People often cut off beetroot greens and throw them away, but these leaves are not only rich sources of vitamins, minerals and phytochemicals, especially betalains, which have a potent anti-inflammatory and detoxification effect, they are also particularly good at increasing alkalinity in the body. (Smokers take note: beetroot greens also help reduce nicotine cravings!) If you choose this Success Booster, add the beetroot greens to your I-Burn Soup when making it before you start your plan, instead of when you are warming up your soup. They should be part of the recipe from the beginning, so the greens get cooked along with the other greens in the soup.

What You Need:

- Fresh beetroot greens, preferably still attached to the beetroots before use. Beetroot greens last only for a day or two after cutting, so use them right away. Look for crisp, fresh, deeply coloured greens that aren't wilted.

Step by Step:

1. Cut the beetroot greens from the beetroots, trim away the long stems, wash, and pat dry. Reserve the beetroots to eat separately (they are an ingredient in several of the I-Burn recipes, including Hummus Coleslaw and recipes that include roasted vegetables).

2. Chop the leaves and add 225g to your I-Burn Soup when you add the other greens.

Deep Breathing

Deep breathing exercises accomplish many of the I-Burn's goals, especially stress management, oxygenation of tissue and increased alkalinity. Deep breathing is an ancient practice. In India, it is called *pranayama*, and it is considered the path to a quiet, calm, enlightened mind. According to this philosophy, a central energy channel runs through the middle of the body, and deep breathing activates the life force within this channel, moving energy throughout the body from top to bottom. This practice is believed to gradually coax the body and mind into a higher state of being. There are many different *pranayama* techniques, but you can start very simply.

When you do these exercises, try not to breathe from your upper chest, and do not move your shoulders as you inhale and exhale. Keep them still and try to fill your lower abdomen with air. This can feel difficult at first, but it is easy to learn with practice. This will help you access a deeper part of your lungs, which will more fully oxygenate your entire body, as oxygen from the lungs moves through the mucosal lining into the bloodstream via tiny capillaries at the ends of the branches of your lungs.

What You Need:
- Nothing other than a quiet spot and a few minutes

Step by Step:
1. Sit on the floor or in a chair with your back straight. Do not lean back on anything, unless you cannot sit straight on your own. Close your eyes and breathe normally for a few seconds.

2. Inhale slowly to a count of approximately 5 seconds. Remember not to move your shoulders and to breathe from your lower abdomen. Exhale slowly to a count of approximately 5 seconds.

3. Inhale slowly to a count of approximately 6 seconds. Exhale slowly to a count of approximately 6 seconds.

4. Repeat, inhaling and exhaling to a count of 7, 8, 9 and 10.

5. Repeat again, but inhale and exhale to a count of 10, then 9, then 8, all the way back down to 5.

6. Breathe normally for a minute or so, until you feel ready to move on with your day.

Epsom Salts Bath

Magnesium sulphate, commonly known as Epsom salts, is a naturally occurring substance composed of two compounds that are essential to our well-being: magnesium and sulphate (or oxidized sulphur). We need magnesium to regulate our enzymes and reduce inflammation, and we need sulphur to create amino acids, digest food and detoxify the body. Because magnesium sulphate can be easily absorbed through the skin, taking a bath is a simple and relaxing way to boost your levels of both essential minerals while also detoxifying.

What You Need:
- 225g Epsom salts
- A warm bath

Step by Step:
1. Add the Epsom salts to the water in your tub.

2. Soak for at least 12 minutes, up to three times per week.

Essential Oils

Essential oils are concentrated liquids made of aromatic compounds from plants. The best essential oils are typically steam-distilled and 100 per cent pure. The essential oils I like for the I-Burn include bergamot, cinnamon, clove, eucalyptus, fennel, rose and thyme. Among their many qualities, these have properties that support kidney function, have antibacterial and antifungal effects, and are tonics to reactive nerves. Add a few drops of any or a combination of these oils to a relaxing bath (including the Epsom salts bath in this chapter—two Success Boosters in one!). You can also use them for a targeted self-massage.

What You Need:
- Bergamot, cinnamon, clove, eucalyptus, fennel, rose and/or thyme essential oil
- Cold-pressed raw coconut oil or all-natural massage oil

Step by Step:
1. Add a few drops of essential oil (or a combination, for example, of cinnamon and clove, or bergamot and rose) to a small scoop of coconut oil or a palmful of massage oil, and mix together with your hands or in a small bowl.

2. Massage this mixture into any areas where you have cellulite, to help activate and dissolve subcutaneous fat. Besides areas of pronounced cellulite (those lumpy spots), focus on the lower back around your waistline, your upper arms and the areas that tend to swell when you are retaining fluid, such as wrists, hands, knees and ankles.

Flower Essences

Flower essences, sometimes called flower remedies, are gentle, safe, benign natural healing essences made from flowers. They are non-toxic and treat emotions rather than physical symptoms, so they are an excellent way to address the emotional imbalances in each of the plans. For the I-Burn, the remedies I like are Rescue Remedy or Five-Flower Formula. Both are combinations of flower essences that were made to soothe reactivity and create more calm.

What You Need:
- Rescue Remedy (Bach Flower Remedy) or Five Flower Remedy (Flower Essence Services)

Step by Step:

There are several ways to use flower remedies. You can take 10 drops in 225ml water and sip throughout the day. You can dab them on your pulse points like perfume, or you can put them in a spray bottle with spring water and mist them onto your skin. You can also mix 20 drops into 55ml of neutral unscented skin cream. Taste it, touch it, smell it and it will help you.

Meditation

Meditation is an ancient practice with super contemporary benefits. It can do great things for your blood pressure, your heart rate and especially your relaxation response, quelling the release of destructive stress hormones. I like it for all three of the *Burn* plans, and you will see that I have included a particular meditation technique best suited for each plan. For the I-Burn, I like mindfulness meditation, because it has been shown in several recent studies (including a 2014 study from Europe published in *Psychoneuroendrocrinology*) to reduce reactivity and stress, and also to suppress the expression of the genes RIPK2 and COX2 and the histone deacetylase genes, which are involved in triggering inflammation in the body. An additional perk: the regular practice of meditation will also help your brain work better—and I bet we can all use a little of that!

Mindfulness meditation is a technique for focusing on an object, to train the mind to observe the present moment neutrally, without reactivity and an automatic stress response. Here's how to do it.

What You Need:
- Nothing but a quiet place to sit comfortably
- Optional: a cool comfy meditation cushion or meditation bench
- Optional: an app for your phone that times your meditation and rings soothing chimes or gongs to alert you when to start or finish (search for "meditation apps")

Step by Step:
1. Sit quietly with your back straight. Don't lean against anything unless you must in order to be comfortable. Cross your legs, fold

them under you or sit in a chair with both feet flat on the ground. Set a timer for five minutes for your first try. If you are already a meditator, you can do 10, 15 or even 20 minutes. If not, this can be a goal for you to work up to, if you like meditation and decide to stick with it after you are through with your three-day plan.

2. Take a few quiet calming breaths. Focus on how that feels. Notice the feel of the breath coming in and going out. How does it feel in your nostrils? In your throat? What parts of your body move with your breath? Examine the sensations in as much detail as you can. If your mind wanders, bring it back to noticing the sensation of breathing as soon as you notice it has strayed.

3. After you've done this for a while and you feel like you want to focus on something else, focus on how your whole body feels. What do you notice the most? Does a part of you feel noticeable at the moment? Does something feel good, or does something hurt? Turn your attention to this sensation, but do not attach any opinions or reactions to it. Just observe, as if it were happening to someone else. Stay with this until your time is up.

4. When the timer goes off, take a few deep, calming breaths, get up slowly, and move on through your day with a calm, non-reactive mind. The more you do this, the less reactive you will become, and the more inflammation-reducing effects you will enjoy.

Reflexology

Reflexology is a way to heal and detoxify your body by applying varying degrees of pressure to specific areas of the hands, feet and ears that are believed to be reflex points, or energy points connected to other areas of the body. Pressing and massaging these points is thought to help activate, energize and heal the area to which that point is associated. For I-Burn purposes, we want to activate the kidneys, bladder and lymphatic system, for more efficient detoxification. Many massage therapists are trained in reflexology and can activate these points for you, but you can also do it yourself. The following diagram shows where these points are on the foot. You can also use the I-Burn essential oils on the points shown—combining Success Boosters really ups the effects of both.

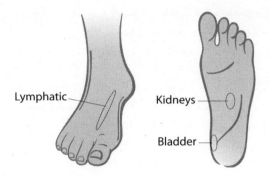

What You Need:

- A quiet spot and an unoccupied pair of hands (or a reflexologist or friend willing to rub your feet!)

Step by Step:

1. Sit down in a relaxed position. Take off your shoes and socks. Take your foot into your hands.

2. To stimulate and activate your lymphatic system, gently but firmly rub your thumb up and down the top of your foot, from the base of the space between your big toe and second toe down about 7.5cm, as indicated in the diagram. Rub this area up and down.

3. Turn your foot over so you are looking at the sole. To stimulate and activate the kidneys, press and rub the spot in the centre of your foot about an inch inside the arch, as indicated in the diagram.

4. To stimulate and activate the bladder, press and run your finger in a line down from the kidney spot along the inside edge of the arch to the top of the heel, as indicated in the diagram.

5. Repeat on the other foot.

SUPPLEMENT BOOST FOR THE I-BURN

Many additional vitamins, minerals and other supplements can improve the work you are doing on the I-Burn, but don't just take any supplements. Many are cheap and contain adulterated ingredients as well as relatively ineffective versions of the compounds. Be sure you buy from a reputable company that uses the highest-quality, unadulterated ingredients. Because this is such a problem in a relatively unregulated supplement industry, I have manufactured a line of *Burn* supplements that are pure and free of adulteration. You certainly don't have to buy them, but if you want to go with a good source, this is one option. These are the supplements I recommend for the I-Burn (you can find them at shophayliepomroy.com):

- Metabolism Multi: Targeted Multivitamin Mineral Blend
- Metabolism AI: Targeted Anti-Inflammatory Blend

INTENSE BOOSTS

Infrared Sauna

Although the term *infrared* may sound space-agey to you, infrared saunas are gentle and operate at a lower heat than typical dry saunas. Instead of using heated rocks like a dry sauna, infrared saunas use infrared heaters and infrared light to produce radiant heat that your body absorbs. Sweating in an infrared sauna increases your metabolism and circulation, and I like it for the I-Burn because it is a gentle way to release fluid and impurities through the skin. It is a comforting but compelling way to detox. The only caution I would give you is not to let yourself get overheated and to drink plenty of water before, during and after your sauna time, as would apply to any sauna or heat therapy. If you become uncomfortable or dizzy, leave the sauna and relax until you feel better. Unless you are heat-sensitive, you shouldn't have any problem with an infrared sauna. If you start slowly and work your way up to more time as you get used to the experience, you should remain comfortable and still get all the circulation-enhancing and detoxification benefits.

What You Need:
- An infrared sauna in your home or a friend's house or at a community health centre, gym, or spa

- Plenty of water to drink before, during and after
- Towels to sit on and for wiping off sweat

Step by Step:
1. Take a warm bath or shower before entering the sauna.

2. Enter the sauna and sit on towels, for 10 minutes to start, working up to 30 minutes if you continue to use the sauna on a regular basis (the amount of time will depend on the sauna's heat and your personal tolerance—if you start to feel at all uncomfortable, dizzy or nauseated, leave the sauna). Wipe off sweat as needed.

3. After the sauna, sit for 10 to 20 minutes before showering to allow your body to cool down.

4. Rinse off the perspiration with cool-to-warm water.

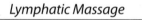

Lymphatic Massage

I'm a proponent of many types of massage, but the type I like best for the I-Burn is a lymphatic massage. This gentle technique involves invigorating lymphatic circulation and drainage by massaging over the lymph nodes and then manually manipulating the lymph toward the kidneys, where it can dump its toxins for removal. It is a commonly prescribed therapy for people who have had to have lymph nodes removed and who are prone to swelling because of this, but it can also benefit anyone whose lymphatic flow is slow and sluggish, who is retaining water and/or who is accumulating subcutaneous fat.

Lymphatic massage feels gentle and relaxing, but afterward you will notice a big shift. Over the next few days, swelling tends to go down dramatically so that you see more of your ankles and wrists again and notice more definition all over your body. It's not just about looking better, however. Lymphatic massage is a powerful way to assist the body in detoxification.

What You Need:

- A massage therapist, doctor, nurse or other healthcare professional who has been trained and certified in lymphatic massage. Ask your doctor or local massage therapist for referrals
- About an hour of your time

Step by Step:

Make an appointment, relax and enjoy! Afterward, drink lots of water to help your lymphatic system move everything that has been stimulated out of your body.

Rebounding (Mini Trampoline)

Rebounding is a low-impact exercise that improves the flow of the lymphatic system by stimulating all muscle groups at once. It is an efficient lymphatic system detoxifier, and it's also great exercise, building muscles and strengthening bones. It involves bouncing on a personal-sized trampoline. The trampoline reduces the potentially damaging impact of jumping on your joints and connective tissue, so you can jump for an extended period of time without injury. Plus, it's fun!

What You Need:

- A rebounder, which is just a mini-trampoline. You can purchase these at most sporting goods stores. If you are a bit unsteady on your feet or have balance issues, get a rebounder that comes with a bar to hold on to while you jump.

Step by Step:

1. Step on the rebounder.

2. Jump. Begin slowly and gently until you get used to it. Vary your movements—jump low, jump high, even twist and dance around. Have fun with it. Try it to music, or do it while you watch TV. Start with shorter sessions of about 5 minutes. If you continue using the rebounder, work up to 20 minutes at a time, as you get fitter and stronger.

D-BURN SUCCESS BOOSTERS

D-Burn Success Boosters are designed to do one or more of the following:

- Calm the digestive tract
- Calm and clear the lungs and respiratory system
- Heal the mucosal lining
- Encourage vasodilation to dissolve and release yellow fat
- Stimulate excretion from the colon
- Reduce intestinal gas, bloating and flatulence
- Remedy constipation and/or diarrhoea

EXERCISE BOOST

On any day you choose to exercise, I prefer you do so before 2:00 p.m. for maximum benefit, because this is when your body is most receptive to vigorous activity, especially the higher-intensity cardio I like you to do on the D-Burn. However, exercising later in the day is better than not exercising at all. One exception: don't exercise within one hour of bedtime. This can be too stimulating and can make sleep difficult. It also works against what your body is naturally trying to do as it slows down and prepares for the repair and rebuilding that happens when you sleep.

Although the Success Boosters you choose are totally up to you, exercise is effective for penetrating and emulsifying the thick, stubborn yellow fat we are trying to blast through with the D-Burn, so I encourage you to include exercise Success Boosters as part of your D-Burn experience.

Vigorous Cardio

Whether it's jogging on a treadmill or outdoors, working out on the elliptical trainer or in a spin class, or doing good old-fashioned aerobics, cardio is the name of the exercise game on the D-Burn plan. The reason is that cardiovascular exercise boosts the ability of your circulatory and lymphatic systems to facilitate the spread of nutrients and the removal of toxins. All of your organs benefit from that, which helps boost the dietary work you do on this plan. For the D-Burn in particular, it strengthens your respiratory system and helps your blood vessels carry oxygen. Choose any type you like, but get your heart rate up and start sweating!

What You Need:
- A supportive pair of exercise shoes

Step by Step:
Do 30 minutes of vigorous cardio, such as brisk walking or jogging outside or on a treadmill, using an elliptical trainer, bicycling, jumping rope, brisk hiking, or taking an aerobics class, spin class, power yoga class, or any other activity that gets your heart pumping. Remember that you may do more than one Success Booster every day, so if you do vigorous cardio three times or even every day during the D-Burn, along with other Success Boosters that interest you, this will only increase the plan's good effects.

D-BURN SMOOTHIE BOOST

Aloe Vera Juice

Aloe vera juice comes from the aloe vera plant, which is known for the gel-like contents of its thick leaves. People often use the gel straight from the plant—just tear off a leaf and rub the gel on a sunburn or abrasion. However, aloe vera juice is equally healing to the insides. You can buy it in juice form. I add it to the D-Burn Smoothie because it heals the mucosal lining and can also help relieve constipation and colitis.

What You Need:
- Aloe vera juice, which you should be able to purchase from a well-stocked health food store, or a hearty and large aloe vera plant

Step by Step:

Add 70ml aloe vera juice to your D-Burn Smoothie. Blend and drink. If you want to use the gel from your own plant, cut off a large leaf with a sharp knife or scissors. Cut away all the green parts and lift the fillet of gel from the centre with the side of a knife. Add this to your D-Burn Smoothie before blending.

D-BURN TEA BOOST

Pau d'Arco Tea

This tea is from the bark of the pau d'arco tree, which comes from the South American rainforest and has long been a folk medicine remedy in Brazil. It has a bitter taste, but when mixed with other teas, it can be pleasant. Pau d'arco has many uses, but I like it for D-Burns because of its antibiotic effect—it is a tonic for intestinal infections and diarrhoea, and it can also treat excess yeast. It also has a clearing effect on the respiratory system, helping to loosen and dislodge phlegm so you can cough it up. It is a traditional remedy for bronchitis. Even if you don't have bronchitis or an intestinal infection, it is still a tonic for the mucosal lining and has antioxidant properties. Buy your pau d'arco tea from a trustworthy source—less ethical companies may be selling false products under this name. You need to steep pau d'arco bark for 8 to 10 minutes to release its medicinal properties, so either boil it ahead of time and add the decoction to your D-Burn Tea in the morning, or make sure you have enough time to let it steep.

What You Need:
- Loose pau d'arco tea or pau d'arco tea bag; you'll need 2 to 3 teaspoons or 1 tea bag per cup
- Tea ball or other device for preparing loose tea, if you aren't using a tea bag
- Boiling water or heated D-Burn Tea

Step by Step:

1. Add 2 to 3 teaspoons of loose pau d'arco tea or 1 tea bag to your prepared and heated D-Burn Tea. Or, if you want to drink this separately, add it to boiling water.

2. Steep the tea leaves for 8 to 10 minutes, then drink.

D-BURN SOUP BOOST

Fennel

Fennel is a delicately sweet licorice-scented and -flavoured vegetable related to celery. It has wispy fronds and a bulb with juicy celery-like stems. I like fennel for the D-Burn because it is good at deflating intestinal gas, thanks to the aspartic acid it contains. It also helps purge phlegm and mucus from the intestine, and the anethole and cineole in fennel have an antibacterial effect that can help with indigestion-related stomach issues such as diarrhoea and heartburn. These compounds also have an expectorant effect, helping to clear the lungs. Fennel contains high levels of vitamin C, folate and potassium, as well as fibre, so it nourishes while encouraging the bowels to move.

What You Need:

- Fresh fennel. Look for crisp and firm bulbs with straight stems and no brown spots. They should look fresh and juicy, not dry and cracked.

Step by Step:

1. Trim the tough ends of the greens and the root from the fennel bulb and rinse the bulb.

2. Coarsely chop the bulb, including the tender green parts and the wispy fronds; add 10g to your D-Burn Soup.

Raw Apple Cider Vinegar

Although there have been all kinds of health claims about vinegar over the years, one thing it works for is stomach upset. Apple cider vinegar has antibiotic properties, and the pectin it contains can relieve stomach cramps, diarrhoea and nausea. It's also soothing for a sore throat and will help drain stopped-up sinuses. If you are on the D-Burn and having any digestive issues, apple cider vinegar is a helpful tonic, but be sure to buy the raw type in health food stores, not the commercial type. Always dilute apple cider vinegar with water. Taking it straight could damage your tooth enamel.

What You Need:
- Raw apple cider vinegar. You can find raw apple cider vinegar at health food stores or in the health food section. Bragg is a dependable brand.

Step by Step:
Measure 1 to 2 tablespoons apple cider vinegar into 225ml of room-temperature water and drink.

Black Walnut Powder

Medicines, dyes and food have all been made from the hull of the black walnut tree for over four thousand years. The black walnut tree contains juglone, a compound toxic to some plants (though others are tolerant) that can have antifungal, antibacterial and antitumour properties for humans and is also traditionally used as an antiparasitic. The hulls contain tannins, which absorb harmful substances in the digestive tract and help the gastrointestinal tract maintain healthy flora. They can also absorb medication, so talk to your doctor if you are on prescription medication and want to try black walnut powder. The powder is a traditional remedy for constipation, and it is an excellent source of iodine, sulphur, magnesium, potassium, vitamin C, zinc and other micronutrients. Warning: if you are allergic to tree nuts, avoid black walnut powder.

What You Need:
- Powdered black walnut hulls, available from most herbal supply stores. You could also buy this in a tincture form to add to water.

Step by Step:
Measure ½ to 1 teaspoon powder and add to water. You can take it up to three times per week and up to two weeks at a time. Black walnut powder is not meant for long-term use, so it's best to take it only while doing the D-Burn. If you have taken black walnut powder every day for two weeks, take at least two weeks off before trying it again. It has not been studied for long-term use and while it has great short-term benefits, it may cause stomach upset if you use it for more than two weeks. For the tincture, follow the instructions on the bottle.

Cultured/Fermented Vegetables

Cultured vegetables such as sauerkraut, kimchi and lacto-fermented pickles are excellent sources of probiotics, which help the gastrointestinal tract heal and stay strong. These are incredibly nourishing for your gut bacteria and also delicious. You can purchase cultured vegetables from most stores, but it's also easy to make your own using one of several methods. The easiest way only requires salt, water and clean glass jars. You can also add a starter culture, which you should be able to purchase from your local health food store. Use the kind you would to make kefir or yogurt. This will speed up the fermentation process, but it's not strictly necessary. Start by eating small amounts of fermented veggies to see how they agree with you, and increase amounts as your taste and tolerance for them increases.

What You Need:
- The vegetables of your choice, chopped or shredded into smaller pieces—good choices are cabbage, green beans, courgettes, cauliflower, sliced carrots and, of course, cucumbers

- Large, sterilized wide-mouth glass preserving jars with lids—enough to hold the amount of vegetables you want to culture
- Filtered water
- Sea salt, approximately 3 tablespoons for every 2.25kg of vegetables
- Optional: kefir grains or freeze-dried starter culture

Step by Step:

1. Place the vegetables and salt in a large bowl and toss to coat. Stir in the starter culture, if using.

2. Pack the veggies into a preserving jar, leaving 5cm of head space.

3. Add filtered water, just enough to barely cover the vegetables. Cover the jar and leave it on the counter at room temperature for three to ten days. Taste periodically with a clean spoon—when the liquid tastes tangy, your cultured veggies are ready. The longer it ferments, the tangier it will get, so taste to find the level of tartness you prefer.

4. When they are finished, keep the jar in the refrigerator. The veggies should keep for four to six weeks and will continue to ferment slowly in the refrigerator.

Enjoy your fermented veggies with any meal, plain, gently heated or added to a salad.

Detox Bath with Pau d'Arco Tea

Pau d'arco bark not only is great for making a tea but can also be used for detox baths. Used externally, pau d'arco is a potent antifungal, inhibits yeast growth and heals the skin. However, the detox bath is also a good way to heat the body, increasing circulation to those stubborn fatty areas. It is also soothing and relaxing, which reduces stress and promotes a healing environment in the body. Because your skin is the largest organ of elimination, this treatment helps draw out toxins and increase systemwide circulation, which is in turn healing to the mucosal lining. Remember to buy your pau d'arco tea from a trustworthy source.

What You Need:
- Loose pau d'arco bark
- A cloth tea bag or metal tea ball

Step by Step:
1. Place the bark into the tea bag or tea ball.

2. Hang the bag/ball under the tap and fill the bathtub with warm-to-hot water.

3. Soak in the tub for up to an hour.

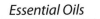

Essential Oils

Essential oils are concentrated liquids made of aromatic compounds from plants. The best essential oils are typically steam-distilled and 100 per cent pure. The essential oils I like for the D-Burn include oregano, nutmeg, peppermint, cardamom and clove. These have various effects. For example, oil of oregano has an expectorant effect on the lungs and also promotes the secretion of digestive enzymes, even when used topically. Nutmeg has properties that deflate gas and soothe indigestion. Peppermint oil is soothing to the digestive tract, and cardamom encourages healthy bile production. Clove oil has a calming effect on the lungs and is a natural remedy for bronchitis and sinusitis. It's also a remedy for hiccups, nausea and gas. Also, essential oils are simply soothing and pleasant; they evoke relaxation and a positive feeling, and this promotes healing in the body, which will impact the mucosal lining. The very best way to promote healing is to create a healing environment in the body, and essential oils are one way to help do this. Add a few drops of any or several of these oils to a relaxing bath. You can also use it for a targeted D-Burn self-massage that focuses on your belly, to help relax and also activate and increase circulation to those fatty areas.

What You Need:
- Oregano, nutmeg, peppermint, cardamom and/or clove essential oil
- Cold-pressed raw coconut oil or all-natural massage oil

Step by Step:
1. Add a few drops of essential oil (or a combination, for example, of oregano, nutmeg and peppermint oils) to a small scoop of coconut oil or a palmful of massage oil, and mix together with your hands or in a small bowl.

2. Massage this mixture into your belly or torso area, wherever you are collecting that thick, hard, yellow fat.

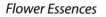

Flower Essences

More than any other Success Booster, flower essences address the emotional component of healing. When you need the D-Burn, you tend to be stuck. You might be having issues with stagnation, indecisiveness or an inability to get moving, and you may also be feeling stubborn and stuck in your ways. My two favourite flower essences to address this are Chestnut Bud, which is good for stagnation and indecision, and Agrimony. I especially like Agrimony for getting you unstuck when you can't seem to get out of a tense emotional space. It will pop your emotions like a balloon. This can be useful when you feel reactive or unreasonably angry, or you just can't break out of a negative head space, but fair warning: use this at home when you are ready to be emotionally unstuck and have a box of Kleenex with you. It's all going to come pouring out, baby, and then it's all going to be OK.

What You Need:
- Chestnut Bud or Agrimony flower remedies (Bach Flower Remedies)

Step by Step:
There are several ways to use flower remedies. You can take 10 drops under the tongue, or mix them with a small amount of water and take

by the spoonful or in a small glass. You can dab them on your pulse points like perfume, or you can put them in a spray bottle with spring water and mist them onto your skin. You can also mix 20 drops into 55ml of neutral unscented skin cream. Taste it, touch it, smell it and it will help you.

Meditation

Meditation is great for everyone, but different types are useful for different kinds of issues. For the D-Burn, I like mantra meditation. The vibration from repeating the mantra is physically soothing to the lungs and even the digestive tract, but even more importantly, it creates a calm, centred environment that is highly conducive to healing. This helps the body restore and repair digestive and respiratory issues and more smoothly release toxins coming out of the yellow fat that you are burning on the D-Burn.

What You Need:
- Nothing but a quiet place to sit comfortably, where your chanting won't disturb others or make you feel self-conscious
- Optional: a cool comfy meditation cushion or meditation bench
- Optional: an app for your phone that times your meditation and rings soothing chimes or gongs to alert you when to start or finish (search for "meditation apps")

Step by Step:
1. Sit quietly with your back straight. Don't lean against anything unless you must in order to be comfortable. Cross your legs, fold them under you or sit in a chair with both feet flat on the ground.

2. Take a few quiet calming breaths. Now, I want you to think of a word that makes you feel calm. It can be any word you want. If you are into yoga, maybe you will choose *Om*, a mystical Indian syllable that is said to imitate the sound of the vibration of the universe. Or if that's too esoteric or just not you, think of something else. I think one-syllable words work best. Some suggestions: *love, peace, calm, soft, kind, clear, strong, health, life.*

3. In a quiet, steady voice, repeat the word in a slow rhythm, holding out the vowel for about 5 seconds with each repetition. When distractions and unrelated thoughts enter your head (which they will), gently push them aside and go back to your word. Focus on the sound of it, and how it feels in your body as you speak it.

4. Continue for 5 minutes the first time, and gradually work up, minute by minute, until you are meditating for 15 to 20 minutes per session.

5. You can do this just once during the D-Burn, or do it every day (remember, you can always choose more than one Success Booster each day). Ideally, you will keep your meditation habit after you're done with the D-Burn. The best results come from meditating for about 15 to 20 minutes twice a day, once in the morning and once in the evening, but even once a day will make a big impact on your brain function and stress management (which in turn benefits everything else you are trying to do in your life, like work effectively, sustain better relationships, lose weight or whatever else you're living through).

Neem Oil

Neem oil has been used in India for cosmetics and medicine for over six thousand years. Made from the nuts of the neem tree, the oil inhibits the growth of bacteria, fungus, parasites and viruses. It's also a potent antiseptic that repels biting insects that spread disease, such as mosquitoes and ticks. It heals and increases circulation to the skin. I like neem oil for the D-Burn because it is so therapeutic and soothing for the skin. This helps the skin work more effectively as a detox organ. Because so much of what we do on the D-Burn is designed to heat up the body to penetrate and emulsify fat, having strong functional skin with good blood flow helps get rid of everything you will be sweating out.

What You Need:
- Neem oil. It is naturally semi-solid; it is fine if you find neem oil that is blended with another oil. In fact, it makes it easier to pour.

Step by Step:

Add 20 to 25 drops of neem oil to about 225ml of a carrier oil (such as coconut oil, grapeseed oil, sesame oil) or lotion. Rub it into your pelvic area and all over your stomach area.

Oil Pulling

Oil pulling is an ancient Ayurvedic treatment that detoxifies the mouth and gums. Maintaining oral health is one of the most important ways to prevent illness that can quickly spread throughout the body via the circulatory system. Oil pulling also stimulates digestive enzymes as it pulls toxins from the body via the mouth. The mouth is the gateway to digestion, and digestion starts here. Oil pulling will help keep this area healthy and clean.

What You Need:
- 1 to 2 teaspoons of raw, cold-pressed oil, such as coconut, sesame or sunflower, preferably organic

Step by Step:
1. Put the oil into your mouth.

2. Swish it around your mouth for 20 minutes.

3. Spit out the oil; do not swallow it, as it contains bacteria from between your teeth that we want to get rid of.

4. Rinse your mouth with warm water. Some people like to use salt water for this, as they think it cleanses the oil more effectively. You can try this, but I find that regular water works just fine as well.

5. Brush as usual.

Olive Leaf Extract

Made from the leaves of olive trees, this extract contains oleuropein, a powerful polyphenol with anti-inflammatory properties that stimulates the immune system and reduces abdominal bloating and gas. Olive leaf extract also treats cold symptoms, pneumonia and chronic fatigue as well as gastrointestinal infections. I especially like it because it facilitates the flow of blood through the circulatory system, which helps with fat incineration.

What You Need:
- Olive leaf extract in capsules standardized to 10 per cent to 15 per cent oleuropein or in 500-mg to 700-mg dosages

Step by Step:
Take one capsule with a full glass of water, twice per day during or after a meal, or according to package directions.

Reflexology

Reflexology is a healing technique that operates on the principle that areas on the feet correspond energetically to every major organ and system in the body. Massaging and applying pressure to the correct area on the foot will help stimulate, activate and heal that area of the body. For the D-Burn, I recommend rubbing and massaging the spots that relate to the lungs, chest and large intestine. See the following diagram. If you use D-Burn essential oils in your reflexology foot massage, you'll get even more bang for your booster buck.

What You Need:
- A quiet spot and an unoccupied pair of hands (or a reflexologist or friend willing to rub your feet!)

Step by Step:
1. Sit down in a relaxed position. Take off your shoes and socks. Take your foot into your hands.

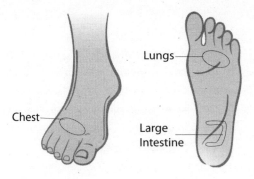

Lungs

Chest

Large Intestine

2. To stimulate and activate your respiratory system, gently but firmly rub your thumb across the top of your foot, beneath your toes, as indicated in the diagram.

3. Turn your foot over so you are looking at the sole. To stimulate the lungs, press and rub just under your toes, as indicated in the diagram.

4. To stimulate and activate the large intestine, press and run your finger in a backward C from the centre of your foot to the outside edge, down along that edge and across again, as indicated in the diagram.

5. Repeat on the other foot.

Soaking Nuts, Seeds, Grains and Legumes

Nuts and seeds are a delicious and easy source of protein, but they also can contain antinutrients that inhibit their proper digestion. Grains and legumes also contain some of these antinutrients. These are all meant to prevent a seed from sprouting prematurely, but they can have an unpleasant digestive effect in the human body. By soaking nuts, seeds, grains and legumes before eating them, you are essentially beginning the sprouting process, even if you don't produce a visible sprout. This reduces the enzyme inhibitors that make these nutritious foods difficult on the digestive system. This also increases the enzyme content. You are essentially turning these seeds into little bundles of potential plant energy, filled with the enzymes they need to grow, and you need to digest them. If you can't find sprouted nuts, seeds, grains and legumes, soaking is easy to do, and I recommend anyone do this whenever they can, but this is important on the D-Burn, when we are honing and facilitating digestion. Note: unless you plan to dehydrate or freeze what you soak, only prepare enough for the recipe you will be making the next day. Soaked food doesn't keep well.

What You Need:
- Nuts, seeds, grains or legumes you plan to eat and/or use in a recipe
- Sea salt
- Filtered water, enough to cover your nuts/seeds/grains/legumes plus about one inch
- Optional: oven or dehydrator

Step by Step:
1. Put the nuts, seeds, grains or legumes in a glass jar or glass bowl. Add about a teaspoon of sea salt. Loosely cover the jar or set a dinner plate on top of the bowl. Put it in a room-temperature spot out of the way and let it sit for 4 to 24 hours. I like to set things out to soak in the evening. The following evening, they are ready to dry or use in a recipe.

2. After 4 to 24 hours, drain and rinse in a colander. Eat or use.

Note about nuts and seeds in particular: soaked nuts and seeds will be softer and chewier than what you are used to. You might like this, or you might prefer to dry your nuts and seeds in a dehydrator or in a very low oven until crunchy. You can also store these in snack-sized or recipe-sized portions in the freezer. Spread them out on paper towels to dry and freeze or dehydrate within 24 hours. To dehydrate using your oven, set it on the lowest setting (75°C/170°F or lower). Spread the nuts, seeds, grains or legumes out on a rimmed baking sheet. Stir every hour or so until the nuts are crispy (depending on air conditions and the heat of your oven, this could take from 4 to 12 hours). Remove when they have reached the desired level of crunchiness.

SUPPLEMENT BOOST FOR THE D-BURN

The supplements perfect for enhancing your D-Burn efforts target your digestion, to repopulate your intestine with good bacteria and give your body a digestive boost with digestive enzymes. Again, this is an optional boost. Since I know what is in my supplements, I'm comfortable recommending them. But you can also buy from a trusted source of your own. These are the supplements I recommend for the D-Burn (you can find them at shophayliepomroy.com):

- Metabolism Multi: targeted Multivitamin Mineral Blend
- Metabolism Digestive Enzyme: unleash Micronutrients from Your Food
- Metabolism Pro-Biotic: promotes Healthy Gut Flora

INTENSE BOOSTS

Dry Sauna

Saunas were developed by ancient Scandinavians to promote relaxation and wellness in a harsh climate, but many cultures have customs that involve sweating for detoxification. Sweating is one of the best and easiest ways to eliminate toxins stored in the body. Sauna use has been shown to reduce a host of illnesses, such as chronic pain, rheumatoid arthritis and chronic fatigue syndrome. It also facilitates recovery after colds, the flu and childbirth. Sauna promotes detoxification by activating your body's monocytes, a type of white blood cell that plays a crucial role in boosting your immunity. Because of the lack of humidity (the only moisture in a dry sauna occurs if you are able to pour some water on the hot rocks, which is neither necessary nor always possible, say in a health club setting), dry saunas are also more vasodilating than infrared saunas. The heat is more intense, which helps heat up and penetrate the thick yellow fat. Although some people put dry saunas in their homes, they are most usually available at gyms or health clubs or at local recreation centres and community centres by the swimming pool. You may also find them in hotels when you are travelling.

What You Need:
- Access to a dry sauna
- Towels
- Plenty of water to drink for hydration

Step by Step:
1. Sit in the sauna for 8 to 15 minutes. Drink plenty of water before, during and after.

2. Exit the sauna, rest for a couple of minutes, and then enter a cool shower or pool slowly.

3. Re-enter the sauna and repeat the cycle as often as you like and feel able to.

4. Leave the sauna if you feel ill or lightheaded. Once you work up to it, you can stay in the sauna for up to 20 minutes at a time.

Hot Stone Massage

Hot stone massage is another form of heat therapy that is perfect for the D-Burn because the heat penetrates the skin and stubborn fat, helping to activate and liquefy it for removal by the digestive system. The therapist places hot stones on the body before massaging, which also enhances the massage and makes for a more potent detoxification effect afterward.

What You Need:
- A massage therapist with training and equipment for hot stone massage

Step by Step:
You will lie on a table and the massage therapist will put warm stones on your back in particular areas. It feels amazing, if the massage therapist is good at this type of massage. Be sure to say something if the stones feel too warm for your personal tolerance.

Chlorophyll is not just for plants. Humans can benefit from it greatly as well, and fresh wheatgrass is the best source for its potent, plant-powered healing. Chlorophyll is antiseptic, antibacterial and anti-inflammatory, and it detoxifies the liver, regulates blood sugar and improves feelings of wellness. It is also a potent enzyme delivery system, enhancing your body's ability to easily digest the food you eat. On top of being packed with chlorophyll, wheatgrass also has high levels of protein, vitamin E, magnesium, phosphorus and many other essential nutrients. One study at Memorial Sloan Kettering Cancer Center found positive results when using wheatgrass to treat ulcerative colitis.

Some people can't take the very strong taste of wheatgrass shots, and it even gives some people a stomach ache. If that's you, no need to choose this one, but if you can handle it, then the benefits are immense. Some people add a wheatgrass shot to fresh juice, to make it easier to take, and this is also a fine way to get that chlorophyll. If you are gluten-intolerant, never fear—wheatgrass has not yet developed the trouble-causing proteins in wheat. Some very sensitive people, such as those with severe celiac disease, may want to avoid wheatgrass, just in case.

What You Need:
- A health food store or gym that sells wheatgrass shots, or your own wheatgrass and juicer (it's much easier to buy them, though—some stores sell them frozen in 50 to 110g portions)

Step by Step:
Wheatgrass can be bitter or intensely grassy, and some people don't like the taste. This is why we call them shots! Pour just 55ml in a shot glass, and bottoms up! You'll get a bit of a jolt but a ton of health benefits.

H-BURN SUCCESS BOOSTERS

H-Burn Success Boosters are designed to do one or more of the following things:

- Address imbalance and dysfunction in the pituitary, thyroid and hypothalamus glands, as well as the liver
- Stimulate detoxification in the body, especially of hormone-disrupting toxins such as heavy metals and plastic residues, as well as environmental chemicals
- Work in the body as an antiviral
- Incinerate stubborn hormone-induced white fat
- Break through the most stubborn of weight loss plateaus
- Balance hormones

EXERCISE BOOSTS

H-Burn Exercise Bundle

While exercise can be a one-day affair for the other plans, the H-Burn is different. When you exercise, I want you to do an H-Burn *exercise bundle*. Do each of these H-Burn exercises on three consecutive days. Remember, if you do one, you *must* do them all, because on the H-Burn, we are working hard to re-establish a rhythm in the body that has been lost because of hormonal imbalance. Cycling through a range of exercises in a predictable way not only will help establish this rhythm but is the most effective way to really shake things loose and trigger that white fat to burn. If you do this cycle twice or even three times during the H-Burn, even better. Remember, you can always do more than one Success Booster, and I highly recommend that this cycle be among the ones you choose. This is how the bundle works:

- Day 1: 30 minutes cardio
- Day 2: 20 minutes strength training
- Day 3: 30 to 60 minutes yoga (or other stress-reducing exercise)

For example, you might do cardio on Monday, strength training on Tuesday and yoga on Wednesday. Take a day off and then do it again if you like, on Friday, Saturday and Sunday. You don't need a day off to start a third round, Monday, Tuesday and Wednesday. And voilà, your ten days are done! Here are specific instructions for each exercise:

Cardio

Cardio kicks off the H-Burn bundle because getting the circulation pumping helps get excess hormones moving out of the system. It also has a thermogenic effect on white fat and helps regulate hormone production and reception. Do any activity you enjoy that gets your heart rate up and makes you sweat: aerobics class, brisk walking or jogging, riding a bike, hiking or just running around with your kids.

What You Need:
- A supportive pair of exercise shoes

Step by Step:
1. Do 30 minutes of your favourite cardio. It should be enjoyable and fun so it doesn't cause you more stress.

2. Don't forget to follow it with strength training the next day and yoga the day after.

Strength Training

Compound resistance exercises, such as squats, dead lifts and presses, increase the production of hormones that cause your cells to use glucose more efficiently. These hormonal responses give your body the power to burn fat, improve muscle growth and establish a natural rhythm. For the best results, do a variety of upper-body and lower-body weight lifting using your own body weight as well as weight machines or free weights. Not sure how to use some of those machines? Many gyms have personal trainers you can hire for a single session. Or try an exercise DVD that shows you how to strength-train at home. For the purposes of the H-Burn (and for safety, if you work out unsupervised), stick with lower weights and higher reps. It will have the most potent beneficial hormonal effects. Do not lift weights so heavy that you get to the point where you can't lift them and you are exhausted. This increases stress, and on the H-Burn we want to reduce stress, not make it worse.

What You Need:
- Access to free weights or weight machines at home or a gym
- An experienced lifter or personal trainer (if you have no strength training experience or if you need a spotter), or a DVD that shows you what to do to get an overall workout

Step by Step:
1. Use any combination of dumbbells, kettlebells, barbells and weight machines to perform multi-joint exercises such as overhead presses, squats and biceps curls.

2. Spend about 20 minutes lifting without pausing for more than 1 minute between each exercise.

3. Don't forget to do yoga the next day!

Yoga and Other Stress-Reduction Techniques

The H-Burn is a time for relaxing, gentle yoga or any other exercise that calms you. This could include light stretching on your own, a leisurely walk, or any other gentle exercise class, programme, DVD or anything else that gets you moving but makes you feel calm and good rather than pumped up. If it settles the body and mind, it's good for the H-Burn. I like yoga in particular because it is useful for hormone regulation and rhythm in the body. Yoga helps to reverse the body's natural tendency to store fat under stress, thereby creating excessive hormone production. Yoga helps the liver, gallbladder and thyroid work smarter, not harder. But again, it doesn't have to be yoga, just something you find helps you to relax.

Try Kripalu, Iyengar or any other type of yoga that focuses on relaxation and gentle stretching rather than strength building, high heat or lots of action. Whether you do yoga at home with a book or DVD or freestyle, or you take a yoga class, you will get great H-Burn benefits.

What You Need:
- Loose-fitting clothes
- A yoga mat (also called a sticky mat)
- A yoga book, DVD or class

Step by Step:
It's best to learn yoga first from a qualified teacher who can make sure you are doing the movements correctly and can advise you if you have any medical issues. After you have been introduced to the basics, you may really enjoy that regular class or you may choose to work from a DVD or a yoga book. Aim for 30- to 60-minute sessions. If any pose hurts, stop immediately and discuss your form with your teacher. The following yoga poses are good for you on the H-Burn:

- Downward-facing dog
- Shoulder stand
- All sitting poses
- All reclining poses
- All inversions

H-BURN SMOOTHIE BOOST

One Raw Organic Egg

Raw eggs are a nutritional powerhouse, and they're not just for eggnog during the holidays. Egg yolks contain healthy fats, a ton of fat-soluble essential vitamins and good cholesterol, which helps with hormone production. Yolks also have lecithin, a micronutrient responsible for hormone metabolism; it also improves the health of your liver, skin and brain. I like this Success Booster for men with testosterone production or absorption issues. If you are worried about salmonella, know that most healthy people won't be harmed by the occasional raw egg, but I do encourage you to buy organic and from a local source, if possible. This will reduce the chances of contamination. And if a raw egg simply makes you too nervous? Just choose a different Success Booster. No specific boosters are ever required.

What You Need:
- 1 raw organic egg

Step by Step:

Add 1 egg to your morning smoothie. Blend well.

H-BURN TEA BOOST

Essiac Tea

Essiac is a herbal mixture used to make a herbal tisane. Traditionally, it contains rhubarb root, burdock root, sheep sorrel and slippery elm bark, but some formulations have added to this with additional elements, such as kelp, red clover, watercress and blessed thistle. The components of traditional essiac tea each have detoxification properties. Burdock root is an anti-inflammatory that purifies the blood, aids digestion and rejuvenates the liver. Rhubarb root, used for thousands of years in Chinese medicine, is a purgative. Sheep sorrel has antibacterial, antiviral and anti-inflammatory properties; it reduces blood pressure and increases metabolism. Slippery elm bark facilitates mucus production, which can help with detoxification. The combination of these herbs helps liquefy hard, dense fat in the body. Also, you may notice that some of these elements have benefits that we focus on more in the I-Burn and D-Burn. That is intentional in this tea. I like it for the H-Burn because it has such broad-spectrum, dynamic medicinal effects. This helps with balancing all the systems in the body, which is how we address the underlying hormone dysfunction. Fix the system, put the system into balance, establish a rhythm and the hormones will follow.

What You Need:
- Essiac tea bags or loose tea
- Tea ball or other device for preparing loose tea, if you aren't using a tea bag
- H-Burn Tea, reheated, or hot water

Step by Step:

1. Add an essiac tea bag or loose tea into your reheated H-Burn Tea. Or, if you want to drink it separately, add it to hot water.

2. Let it steep for 2 to 3 minutes.

H-BURN SOUP BOOST

Yams

Yams contain phytonutrients that help stabilize and balance hormones. For women, consistently consuming yams improves the body's cholesterol levels and hormones. In the United States and Europe, sweet potatoes are sometimes called yams. Check with your grocer to ensure you're purchasing true yams, which are rich in vitamins C, B6 and potassium. Certain types of yams contain a compound that can mimic oestrogen. These are beneficial when you are having hormonal issues because the phytoestrogens can block the action of excessive oestrogen, helping to restore balance.

Note: to add yams to your soup, you will need to do so when you prepare it before you start the H-Burn, so if you choose this Success Booster, you will need to purchase it before you make your soup.

What You Need:
- 1 yam, peeled and chopped into bite-sized pieces

Step by Step:
Add the yam pieces to your H-Burn Soup along with the other root vegetables when you prepare it initially.

EASY BOOSTS

Alternate Nostril Breathing

Alternate nostril breathing helps make up for the fact that most of us unintentionally favour one nostril over the other while breathing. This practice helps restore balance to the breath, which in turn balances the body. This is an ideal practice for hormone imbalance because balance in any system helps restore balance in all systems. For this reason, alternate nostril breathing also helps restore balance to the emotions, so this is an ideal Success Booster for when you are feeling subject to mood swings or emotional extremes.

What You Need:
- At least three fingers and a nose

Step by Step:
1. Sitting in a comfortable cross-legged position or in a chair with a straight back, rest your right index finger in the centre of your forehead. Breathe normally for a few breaths and relax.

2. Close your right nostril with your thumb.

3. Inhale slowly through your left nostril.

4. Release your right nostril and close your left nostril with your ring finger.

5. Exhale slowly through your right nostril. Now inhale through your right nostril, slowly.

6. Close your right nostril and release your left nostril. Now exhale through your left nostril.

7. Repeat steps 2 to 6 nine times.

8. Breathe normally for a few breaths. Then move on with your day, balanced and relaxed.

9. When you are comfortable with a regular practice of alternate nostril breathing, you can try a more advanced technique. Try holding your breath for 3 to 5 seconds as you switch nostrils, at the top of the inhale and at the bottom of the exhale. To get even more advanced, hold your breath only after the inhale for an energizing effect. Hold only after the exhale for a calming effect.

Black Pepper

Black pepper is a warming spice that helps increase your internal heat and emulsify stubborn white fat. Especially when combined with a diet rich in turmeric (which you are getting every day in your H-Burn Tea), black pepper has been shown to help rid the body of unusable waste hormones, especially those stored in fat. Add it to any food liberally. It's an especially nice addition to your H-Burn Soup. Black pepper is most potent if you grind it yourself, so get the peppercorns and a good grinder and keep it near where you cook.

What You Need:
- Black peppercorns
- Pepper grinder

Step by Step:
Grind pepper into any savoury food. Use liberally, according to your taste preferences.

Chlorella

Chlorella is a freshwater algae. Why would you want to eat algae? Because it is full of great stuff, such as protein, good fats, antioxidants, chlorophyll, vitamins and minerals. It's also a potent detoxifier, especially of heavy metals. It grabs on to them and shuttles them right out the back door. I love chlorella for the H-Burn because its good fats, high nutrient content and detoxification mechanisms all help to regulate and nourish the hormonal system.

What You Need:
- Chlorella tablets or capsules

Step by Step:
The recommended dose is 500 mg of chlorella, taken every morning. If you find that you get a little bit nauseated when you take this much, start with 250 mg and work your way up slowly as your body adjusts.

Dry skin brushing is a wonderful way to reduce bloating and boost the elimination of toxins through the circulatory and lymphatic systems. It's good for you anytime, including on any of the *Burn* plans, but I like it for the H-Burn because it speeds up detoxification. When you start burning hormone-induced fat rapidly, you will be releasing a heavy dose of fat-soluble toxins that will come out wherever they can. Taking advantage of the skin as the largest detoxification organ in the body is a good way to help ease this process, and dry skin brushing is the best way to enhance detoxification through the skin. This takes some of the burden off the liver. Dry skin brushing also increases the flow of blood to the skin, removes dead skin cells and stimulates the nervous system as well as the production of collagen and elastin. This aids in skin cell turnover and more circulation to skin cells, so that crêpey, drapey skin you can get in the presence of hormonal imbalance looks tighter, smoother and younger again. Get in the habit of dry brushing before you shower and you can enjoy the benefits long past the end of your H-Burn plan.

What You Need:
- A natural-bristle brush that is stiff without being overly hard. You can buy brushes designed for dry skin brushing.

Step by Step:
1. Starting at your feet and using gentle, circular motions, brush your skin, moving toward your heart.

2. Move up your legs, up and down your torso and up your arms, from fingertips to shoulders.

3. Shower when finished.

Essential Oils

The essential oils I like for the H-Burn include sage, basil, ylang-ylang, geranium and frankincense. These are useful for balance. They have a range of benefits but also address many H-Burn issues. Sage is good for fatigue, anxiety, and PMS and menopausal issues. Basil is useful for depression and as an aphrodisiac, if you feel like your sex drive needs a boost. Ylang-ylang has a pleasant scent that helps with mood swings and nervousness. Geranium is rejuvenating and a good remedy for fatigue, while frankincense is calming and a good remedy for anxiety and as an aid to meditation. Smell them as needed by putting a drop on the back of your hand, or use them to massage any new areas of fat you didn't use to have, such as belly fat or saddlebags.

What You Need:
- Sage, basil, ylang-ylang, geranium and/or frankincense essential oil
- Cold-pressed raw coconut oil or all-natural massage oil

Step by Step:
1. Add a few drops of essential oil (or a combination, for example, of sage and basil, or ylang-ylang and frankincense) to a small scoop of coconut oil or a palmful of massage oil, and mix together with your hands or in a small bowl.

2. Massage this mixture into any areas where you have hormone-induced white fat, such as around your rib cage; on the outside of your thighs, neck, knees or waistline; or any other atypical lumpy spots. Or, just rub it everywhere—focusing on your entire body will help your body detox through the skin and help you feel more balanced.

Flower Essences

Flower essences address your emotional issues, which is important for the H-Burn, when your moods may feel completely out of whack and extreme. Many flower remedies address extreme moods, but the two I like for the H-Burn are Gorse and Impatiens. Gorse is a great balancer, helping you find the space between light and dark. If you feel wildly joyful one moment and hopelessly depressed the next, try Gorse to lift you back into that middle space. Impatiens is good for irritability, when you want to snap at someone or can't seem to summon your usual level of patience.

What You Need:
- Gorse or Impatiens flower remedies (Bach Flower Remedies)

Step by Step:
There are several ways to use flower remedies. You can take 10 drops under the tongue, or mix them with a small amount of water and take by the spoonful or in a small glass. You can dab them on your pulse points like perfume, or you can put them in a spray bottle with spring water and mist them onto your skin. You can also mix 20 drops into 55ml of neutral unscented skin cream. Taste it, touch it, smell it and it will help you.

Hormone Detox Cocktail

This little gem is a potent cocktail of detoxifying elements that is perfect for the H-Burn. Ditch the morning OJ and have one of these instead for a greatly improved day. Every element helps purge toxins from your system, for more effective hormone production and internal balance.

What You Need:
- Juice of ½ lemon
- 2 tablespoons raw coconut vinegar (a mild, enzyme-rich vinegar available in health food stores and supermarkets with a well-stocked health food section and online)
- 1 tablespoon grapeseed oil

Step by Step:
1. To make one serving, combine the ingredients in a small glass and stir. Drink first thing in the morning.

2. You can store ten days' worth of the cocktail in a glass jar in the fridge. To make this, juice 5 lemons and combine the juice with 300ml raw coconut vinegar and 150ml grapeseed oil in a jar. Shake and refrigerate. Your morning portion is 55ml.

Hydrotherapy (Wet Sock Treatment)

The wet sock treatment, also known as the cold sock treatment, is a powerful circulation-stimulating and system-balancing form of hydrotherapy that is quite simple, if a little weird. When you put cold socks on hot feet, your body will rush to correct this strange situation, sending all the blood to your feet to warm them. This puts your entire circulatory system on high alert as the body seeks to restore your internal homeostasis. Everything starts moving and your immune system kicks in to get toxins out and restore balance. You will wake up feeling great—more balanced and vigorous than you did the night before. This is also an excellent treatment for the first signs of a virus, as well as one of my favourite remedies for hormone-induced sleep issues.

What You Need:
- One pair of cotton socks
- One pair of wool socks
- A foot-soaking bucket

Step by Step:
1. Before bedtime, drench a pair of cotton socks in cold water and then put them in the refrigerator.

2. Fill a bucket with water as hot as you can stand (but not so hot that it will burn you). Get comfortable and soak your feet in the hot water for 15 minutes.

3. As soon as you are done, dry your feet and immediately put on the cold wet socks from the refrigerator. Cover them with the heavy wool socks and go straight to bed.

When you wake up in the morning, your feet will feel warm and dry, and you will feel amazing.

Meditation

Any form of meditation or stress management is good for the H-Burn, but I find visualization most useful. When you are in the throes of hormonal imbalance, your moods can get pretty wacky, your energy can flag and you can start to feel negative, even depressed. Visualization is like taking a mini vacation. In your mind, you go to a place you most want to be, and that is incredibly relaxing and rejuvenating. This also helps balance extreme moods, by invoking an even and calm sensation. When you are walking on a sunny beach, wandering through a flowery meadow or hiking the Alps, it's hard to feel irritated or blue. Extreme moods tend to lead to extreme thinking and negative mental patterns, negative self-talk and pessimism. Visualization directly reverses this, imposing positive mental patterns, and the effects are measurable: you will enjoy lower blood pressure, deeper and more relaxed breathing, and you can even stop the release of stress hormones, all through the power of your imagination. Here's how to do it.

What You Need:
- Nothing but a quiet place to sit comfortably
- Optional: a cool comfy meditation cushion or meditation bench
- Optional: an app for your phone that times your meditation and rings soothing chimes or gongs to alert you when to start or finish (search for "meditation apps")

Step by Step:
1. Sit quietly with your back straight. Don't lean against anything unless you must in order to be comfortable. Cross your legs, fold them under you, or sit in a chair with both feet flat on the ground. Set a timer for 5 minutes or longer. (This meditation is so enjoyable that you may want to start with 10 minutes.)

2. Take a few quiet calming breaths. Now, imagine a place you most want to be right now in this moment. It can be a place you've been before, like a favourite vacation or a place you remember from childhood. Or, make it up—your perfect beach, your perfect woods, your perfect lakefront, your perfect alpine environment.

3. Now, put yourself in the scene. In as much detail as you can, see everything around you: the colour of the sky, the clouds, the ocean, the flowers, the trees, the panoramic view. Or maybe you are in a secluded garden, or a beautiful room in an amazing

house. Notice everything. Populate the scene with the best possible images and beauty.

4. Now use your other senses. What do you hear? The wind in the trees, the sound of the surf, music? What do you smell? Sand, flowers, fresh-cut grass? What do you feel? Soft grass beneath your feet, water washing over your feet, rock or dirt or leaves, silk or velvet or tile? Are you in a warm bath, a cool stream, on the side of a hill, in the middle of the woods?

5. Now what do you do? Let yourself walk, wander, gaze or just sit and stare at the sky. Continue basking in your beautiful spot until the timer goes off. Take a few breaths and move on with your day. Isn't it nice to have just been on vacation?

Milk Thistle Tincture

Not only is milk thistle one of the best natural remedies for liver issues, it also lowers cholesterol, helps insulin resistance and is a potent anti-inflammatory. It aids the liver in flushing environmental toxins and growing healthy, new cells. You are already getting milk thistle in your tea on the H-Burn, but the tincture has an even more potent medicinal effect on the liver. This is also a great Success Booster if you are having significant hot flushes or hormone-based headaches. (Note: milk thistle is related to ragweed, so those with allergies should avoid using it, as should women who are pregnant or nursing.)

What You Need:
- Milk thistle tincture, preferably organic (look for a dry herb strength ratio of 1:1)

Step by Step:
Take 30 drops of milk thistle tincture or extract in 55 to 110ml of water three times per day between meals.

Pectin Powder

Pectin is a soluble fibre that binds with fat-soluble toxins in the GI tract in particular. It likes to surround and carry out hormone-disrupting compounds such as heavy metals, pesticides, plastic residue and other environmental toxins. Pectin also keeps your bowels moving more smoothly and comfortably.

What You Need:
- Pectin powder supplement (gluten-free), such as apple pectin

Step by Step:
Mix pectin powder with 350 to 475ml of water, with dinner.

Pomegranates and Mulberries

These two fruits, both on the H-Burn food list, contain antioxidants that are excellent for neutralizing free radicals in the body. Because they are less common, you might tend to ignore them, so I want to highlight their benefits here and encourage you to try them. Pomegranates and red mulberries contain the phytochemical resveratrol, which promotes healthy oestrogen metabolism. Studies have demonstrated that pomegranates reduce clotting, lower blood pressure and inhibit several hormone-related cancers, such as breast cancer, prostate cancer and colon cancer. Mulberries contain detoxifying fibre, help balance blood sugar, and may have an antidiabetes effect because of phytochemicals called anthocyanins. White mulberries are helpful for blood sugar control and have been used as a remedy for diabetes. A serving of either pomegranate seeds or fresh mulberries (white or red) is 175g. A serving of dried white mulberries is 50g.

What You Need:
- Fresh pomegranates and/or fresh or dried mulberries. Pomegranates are in season in the autumn and winter. Buy the whole fruit or the seeds. Mulberries are not typically sold in stores, but many people grow them and they grow wild in many areas. White mulberries are native to China and grow in zones

4 to 8. Red mulberries are native to the United States and grow wild especially in the eastern half of the country. You can also buy dried white mulberries in health food stores or sections.

Step by Step:
1. You can buy pomegranate seeds, but if you want to extract them yourself, buy a fresh pomegranate. Begin by cutting it in half. Put both halves in a bowl of water, cut side down.

2. Take one of the halves and bend it flat, then pull the seeds and white pith into the water, trying not to squeeze the juice from too many of them.

3. When you have pulled all the seeds into the water, the white pith will float to the top. Throw it away, drain the seeds and store them in the refrigerator. Eat them plain or put them on your salad. Juicy!

Psyllium Fibre

Excess unusable oestrogen pools in the colon, and you want to wash it away before it gets reabsorbed into the bloodstream. A gluten-free, non-wheat-based psyllium fibre is highly efficient at this job. It will keep your bowels moving and keep that excess oestrogen moving on out. Psyllium can also sweep out other toxins that accumulate in the colon. Getting enough fibre in your diet helps keep your bowel movements regular—an important method for removing toxins—but it also absorbs waste hormones that could be reabsorbed by the body if they don't get eliminated.

What You Need:
- Psyllium fibre supplement (wheat-free and gluten-free), in powder or capsule form

Step by Step:
Take the psyllium according to package directions, with a full glass of water with meals and right before bed.

Reflexology, the holistic practice of massaging certain points on the feet that correspond to all the parts and organ systems in the body, is a pleasant and easy therapy that can help activate and detoxify the liver and thyroid. Just rub the right spots on your feet and you can boost the work the H-Burn is doing in your body. For a double boost, use any of the H-Burn essential oils on the reflexology points.

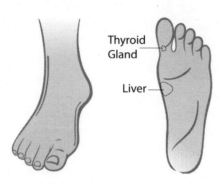

What You Need:
- A quiet spot and an unoccupied pair of hands (or a reflexologist or friend willing to rub your feet!)

Step by Step:
1. Sit down in a relaxed position. Take off your shoes and socks. Take your foot into your hands and turn your foot over so you are looking at the sole.

3. To stimulate the thyroid gland, press just below your big toe, as indicated in the diagram.

4. To stimulate and activate the liver, press and rub about an inch below the ball of your foot, as indicated in the diagram.

5. Repeat on the other foot.

Seaweed and algae are packed with macronutrients and micronutrients such as iron, vitamin C, manganese and iodine. They also lower cholesterol, which helps regulate oestrogen production. Chlorella, in particular, can help your body eliminate lead, dioxin and other industrial toxins.

What You Need:
- Sea vegetables such as nori, dulse, kombu, chlorella and kelp, in whole or powdered form, and/or algae in powdered form

Step by Step:
1. If suggested by the package, soak sea vegetables for 5 to 10 minutes before using.

2. Add 30 to 60g sea vegetables to your H-Burn Soup.

3. Add ½ teaspoon powdered kelp or algae to your H-Burn Smoothie. If you use this regularly, you can work up to 1 teaspoon, but go slowly, as the detoxifying effect is strong (and so is the taste!).

SUPPLEMENT BOOST FOR THE H-BURN

I recommend several supplements for the H-Burn, but look for pure, high-quality brands. I started manufacturing my own when I discovered how many supplements were adulterated with toxins and cheap ingredients. These are the supplements I use for the H-Burn (you can find them at shophayliepomroy.com):

- Metabolism Multi: targeted Multivitamin Mineral Supplement
- Metabolism DIM: targeted Hormone Nutrients
- Metabolism Fatty Acids: the Building Blocks for Healthy Hormones

Castor Oil Packs

Castor oil comes from the seeds of the castor plant, and it is a major source of ricinoleic acid, which has anti-inflammatory properties. Although there are many ways to use castor oil, castor oil packs are excellent for encouraging liver detoxification. The castor oil is absorbed through the skin. Disposable castor oil packs are available for purchase online and in some pharmacies, but you can also make your own. Here's how to use them:

What You Need:
- A 76cm square (approximately) of flannel, wool or felt, which you can fold two or three times, into an approximately 25.5cm square
- Plastic wrap
- An old dish towel or hand towel
- A heating pad
- Old clothes and bedding that you don't mind being stained with castor oil

Step by Step:
1. Saturate a piece of flannel with the castor oil.

2. Place a blanket or towel that can get stained where you want to relax. Get comfortable in clothes that could get stained.

3. Place the oil-saturated cloth over the right side of your abdomen; it should cover from below your rib cage to your hip bone (covering your liver).

4. Cover the flannel with plastic wrap, cover that with another towel, and then put a heating pad on top of that. Turn it on medium or high, depending on your tolerance.

5. Keep the pack on for one hour. Enjoy a book, music or a TV show while letting the castor oil do its work.

6. When you are done, put your oil-soaked cloth in a large plastic zip-top bag for future use. (You can add more oil and use it again for up to two months, but discard it if it turns colour or looks strange to you.) Take a shower to wash the castor oil off your skin.

Clay Bath

Clay is a great way to detox from heavy metals and toxicity from environmental sources. There are several types of clay, and it's important to choose the right sort. The best type of clay for a clay bath is bentonite clay. Avoid any products that contain additives of any kind. You want pure bentonite clay. By detoxing through the skin, you take the burden off the liver, which allows it to be more efficient at neutralizing toxins. Hormone receptors throughout the body also become more efficient when removing toxins that can act like goalies, blocking hormone receptor sites and preventing proper absorption. Drink water before and after your clay bath to facilitate the detox effect.

What You Need:
- Bentonite clay (you can purchase this at most pharmacies and online)
- A fine-mesh drain strainer or hair trap, to catch clay clumps that could clog your drain

Step by Step:
1. Measure 450g of dry, powdered clay.

2. Pour the clay into running bathwater, avoiding any clay dust that gets into the air. Mix the clay in with your hand as the tub fills.

3. Step carefully into the bath and make sure to keep the clay water out of your ears, nose and eyes.

4. Soak for at least 20 minutes. Take a lukewarm shower after the allotted time to wash off the clay and rinse it out of the tub.

Infrared Sauna

The infrared sauna is one of the I-Burn Success Boosters, but I like it here as well because it is so good for detoxification of heavy metals, chemical pesticides and plastics. On the I-Burn, I like you to keep things gentle, but on the H-Burn, I suggest elevating the heat and extending the time for a more intense detoxification experience. You want to sweat a little more and get a little hotter, but certainly don't overdo it. If you feel at all dizzy or nauseated, leave the sauna immediately, and drink plenty of fresh water before, during and after your sauna time.

What You Need:
- An infrared sauna in your home or a friend's house or at a community health centre, gym or spa
- Plenty of water to drink before, during and after
- Towels to sit on and for wiping off sweat

Step by Step:
1. Take a warm bath or shower before entering the sauna.

2. Enter the sauna and sit on towels, for 10 or 15 minutes to start, working up to 30 minutes if you continue to use the sauna on a regular basis (the amount of time will depend on the sauna's heat and your personal tolerance—if you start to feel at all uncomfortable, dizzy or nauseated, leave the sauna). Wipe off sweat as needed.

3. After the sauna, sit for 10 to 20 minutes before showering to allow your body to cool down.

4. Rinse off the perspiration with cool-to-warm water.

Ionic Foot Bath

These systems are a bit pricey, but if you have one, they are excellent for the H-Burn because of their detoxification effects. If you don't have one, you may be able to get access to one at a salon, spa or holistic health clinic. Ionic foot baths can increase alkalinity in your body as they pull acidic chemicals out through your feet. All you have to do is soak your feet in the ionized salt water and relax. The charged ions in the water are thought to bind with toxins having opposite charges and help pull them out.

Note: some sources claim that the brown water that forms during the process is caused by toxins from your feet. This isn't true. It is a result of the ionized water reacting to the salt. I still see a profound detoxifying effect from these machines, however, so I continue to recommend them.

Another note: because of the natural charge in seawater, you can get a similar effect walking in the surf on the beach. I also highly recommend this whenever you have the opportunity.

What You Need:
- An ionic foot bath machine

Step by Step:
1. Prepare the foot bath according to the specific product's instructions, filling it with warm water up to the fill line. Add sea salt. Plug in the machine and turn it on.

2. Put your feet in and relax for about 30 minutes.

3. Turn off the machine and unplug before dumping it out and cleaning it.

4. You can repeat every 3 days on the H-Burn.

Thai Massage Therapy

Thai massage is like a combination of yoga and massage that is wonderful for your hormones. The stretches and sequences of postures centre and ground the body, giving you wonderful long stretches and releasing tight tissue. Happy baby pose, in particular, is great for hormone balancing.

What You Need:
- A massage therapist who specializes in Thai massage

Step by Step:
Go get a massage! Relax and enjoy it. Let it relieve your stress as it increases the circulation in your muscles and tissues.

SUPERVISED SUCCESS BOOSTERS

The Success Boosters in this chapter are the user-friendly ones I pre-scribe to my clients, but I often recommend other therapies that require more professional supervision. I haven't included them in this book because they require the direction of a healthcare practitioner who is qualified and experienced in these areas. If you have a qualified person who can administer these therapies to you, however, and you are inter-ested in trying any of them, talk to your healthcare professional so you can learn more and be sure the therapy is for you. If you still want to go ahead, I believe these therapies can boost your success even further. Each of them can be used in different ways for each of the three *Burn* plans, and they are all effective for detoxification and helping the body heal itself from whatever its issues may be. They are:

Acupuncture
Chelation therapy
Chiropractic
Coffee enemas
Colonics
IV glutathione supplements
IV vitamin C drip
Ozone therapy
Wheatgrass enemas

CHAPTER NINE

Meals in a Flash:
The Burn Recipes

Because *The Burn* is about food, you get to eat a lot of it, and it's all delicious. These are my favourite *Burn* recipes, and they are the ones incorporated into your meal plans. I know you're going to love them, but if you find something in a recipe you cannot eat or do not like, just replace it with something else in the same category on your plan's food list. Replace any vegetable with any other, any fruit with any other, and any protein with any other.

I love to experiment and be creative when I cook, and if you do, I totally relate! However, for *The Burn*, these recipes are not only designed to taste good, but they are also *medicinal in their ingredient makeup*. For this reason, it's essential to make the recipes *exactly as they are written here*. Don't add a grain when there isn't a grain. Don't add more meat or leave it out (unless you are substituting with another protein on your list). Measure the amounts of ingredients, and in particular, *stick with the herb and spice profile*, as this is a crucial aspect of increasing the thermogenic effect of these recipes.

Notice that sometimes a recipe serves more than you will need for that meal; you will be setting a serving aside for a future lunch or dinner. I'll alert you when that happens. Depending on how many people you are feeding and whether you want leftovers, you can always double or even triple any of these recipes. Just remember that you get one portion per meal, and you will stay on track.

So get out your weighing scales and measuring spoons, and enjoy these recipes! They will do amazing things for you if you let them.

I-BURN RECIPES

On the I-Burn plan, the smoothie recipe serves 1 because you will make it fresh every morning. The tea and soup recipes make enough for the entire 3 days. Every lunch recipe serves 1 (double it if you are sharing) and every dinner recipe serves 2. If you are on your own for dinner, cut the recipe in half or save half in the freezer for a future meal after you are finished with the I-Burn.

I-BURN SMOOTHIE

Serves 1

Make this smoothie fresh each morning for maximum micronutrient content.

25g raw walnuts
2 limes, peeled
225ml water
150g ice
50g blueberries (fresh or frozen)
50g cranberries (fresh or frozen)
½ cucumber

¼ avocado
Optional: dash of ground cinnamon
Optional: birch xylitol or pure stevia, if you need more sweetness

Dry-blend the nuts. Add the limes, water, ice, blueberries, cranberries, cucumber and avocado. Blend until smooth. If you need more flavour, you can add a sprinkle of cinnamon and/or a few drops of pure stevia or birch xylitol to taste.

I-BURN TEA
Serves 9 (1 serving = 1 cup)

During the next three days, you will be having a minimum of nine servings of I-Burn Tea. Brew this all at once and then reheat. This tea is truly medicinal, so be sure you let it steep for one to two hours to achieve full potency. I've seen profound effects in my clients' lives from this tea.

2.5 Litres water

9 organic lemons

9 tablespoons dried parsley (do not use fresh—dried works better in this recipe)

3 tablespoons celery seed

¼ teaspoon cayenne pepper

Optional: 2 to 4 drops pure stevia

Pour the water into a pot. Slice the lemons in half, squeeze the juice into the water and drop the rinds into the water. Add the parsley, celery seed and cayenne pepper. Bring to a boil, then let the tea steep for 1 to 2 hours. Filter out the solids and store in the refrigerator. Reheat as needed. If you need a little more sweetness, add a few drops of stevia. Enjoy with breakfast, lunch and dinner.

I-BURN SOUP

Serves 6 (1 serving = 450g)

This is an unlimited food, so this recipe makes more than the 6 servings called for in the meal plan. Eat it between meals as much as you need to if you get hungry, but if you have leftovers, just freeze and enjoy anytime, even after the plan is over.

3.5 Litres water

4 carrots, diced

4 celery stalks, chopped, with leaves

450g chopped greens: spring greens, chard and/or dandelion tops

1 large red onion, chopped

2 sweet potatoes, chopped

350g chopped root vegetables: turnips, parsnips and/or swede

190g fresh or dried shiitake or maitake mushrooms

165g white button mushrooms

200g diced daikon or white radish, root and tops

25g chopped fresh coriander or parsley

2 garlic cloves, peeled

½ teaspoon sea salt, or more, to taste

Combine all ingredients in a stockpot and bring to a boil. Cover and let simmer for 2 hours. Allow to cool. Then purée in a blender, or blend in the pot with an immersion blender. Serve warm, room temperature or chilled. This soup will keep in the refrigerator for up to 5 days, or you can freeze it in individual portions for later use.

I-BURN LUNCHES

SPINACH AVOCADO SALAD WITH WATERMELON

Serves 1

This salad takes only a few minutes to put together, so make it fresh. If you do make it ahead of time to take with you to work, put the dressing in a separate container and dress the salad right before eating.

350g fresh spinach, torn into bite-sized pieces
75g diced watermelon
40g chopped avocado
40g chopped fresh coriander or parsley

25g raw walnuts
Handful of alfalfa sprouts
Juice of ½ lemon
1 tablespoon extra-virgin olive oil
Pinch of black pepper
Pinch of sea salt

Put the spinach in a medium bowl. Top with the watermelon, avocado, coriander, walnuts and sprouts. In a small bowl, whisk together the lemon juice, oil, pepper and salt. Pour the dressing over the salad and toss to coat and mix the ingredients. Enjoy.

HUMMUS COLESLAW

Serves 1

200g shredded cabbage

85g shredded raw beetroots

85g shredded carrots

85g shredded jicama/turnips

85g shredded courgettes

35g raw pine nuts or walnuts

2 tablespoons prepared hummus

1 tablespoon fresh lime juice

Put all ingredients in a medium bowl and toss until the hummus is evenly distributed. If prepared ahead, store in the refrigerator in an airtight container. Do not freeze.

SARDINES AND CUCUMBERS

Serves 1

175g tinned sardines, in olive oil

225g sliced cucumbers

1 teaspoon fresh lemon juice

Sea salt to taste

Combine the sardines with the cucumbers and season with lemon juice and salt. Enjoy this with a pear on the side.

I-BURN DINNERS

DOVER SOLE WITH ROASTED VEGETABLES

Serves 2

*This recipe makes 1.2kg roasted vegetables. Use 600g in this recipe
and set aside the remaining 600g for tomorrow night's dinner,
Roasted Vegetables on Courgette "Pasta".*

350g sliced cabbage

225g sliced carrots

110g sliced white mushrooms

260g diced courgettes

275g diced beetroots

200g sliced tomatoes

4 garlic cloves, diced

4 tablespoons extra-virgin olive oil

2 teaspoons sea salt

Pinch of black pepper

350g Dover sole fillet (or other
     white fish)

Preheat the oven to 220°C/425°F. In a large bowl, toss all the vegetables
with the garlic, oil, salt and pepper. Spread them evenly on a roasting
pan. Roast for half an hour, or until the vegetables are tender and a bit
crisp. In the last 8 minutes of cooking, place the fish on top of the vegetables. Cook for 3 minutes. Flip the fish and cook for an additional 5
minutes. Remove from the oven and serve the sole over the vegetables.

ROASTED VEGETABLES ON COURGETTE "PASTA"

Serves 2

4 medium courgettes

1 tablespoon extra-virgin olive oil

2 garlic cloves, diced

600g leftover roasted vegetables
     from yesterday's dinner

40g raw pine nuts or walnuts

Put the courgettes through a spiralizer or mandoline, or cut them with a
knife into long thin noodle shapes. Heat the oil in a large frying pan over
medium heat. Add the garlic and sauté for about 2 minutes. Add the
roasted vegetables and place the courgette "noodles" on top. Cover the
pan tightly and steam for 5 minutes. Serve hot, garnished with pine nuts.

CAYENNE WATERMELON

Serves 2

160g diced watermelon

Pinch of cayenne pepper

Sprinkle the cayenne pepper over the watermelon and serve.

MEXICAN DINNER SALAD

Serves 2

900g fresh spinach

60g cooked black beans (preferably sprouted, if you can find them; tinned is fine)

200g diced tomatoes

100g diced jicama/turnips (or more to taste)

½ avocado, chopped

40g chopped fresh coriander or parsley

Juice of 2 limes

2 tablespoons extra-virgin olive oil

Sea salt to taste

Pinch of crushed red pepper flakes

Divide the spinach between two salad bowls. Top each with half of the black beans, tomatoes, jicama/turnips, avocado and coriander. Whisk the lime juice and oil together with the salt and red pepper flakes. Divide the dressing between the two salad bowls and serve. Enjoy with the side dish above.

D-BURN RECIPES

On the D-Burn plan, the smoothie recipe serves 1 because you will make it fresh every morning. The tea and soup recipes make enough for the entire 5 days. Every lunch recipe serves 1 (double it if you are sharing) and most dinner recipes serve 4. In those cases, you will have enough for dinner for 2, plus 2 extra servings. You will use one of these later in the week for lunch, as specified, and you will have an extra portion to store in the freezer for another time. If the D-Burn dinner does not require that you save some for a future meal, it will serve 2.

D-BURN SMOOTHIE

Serves 1

Though fresh is best, if you want to make this for the whole plan, take this recipe and multiply its ingredients by five. Pour into single-serving containers and freeze. Then remove, reblend and enjoy.

40g raw pumpkin seeds
1 lemon, peeled
1 teaspoon chia seeds
½ green apple, cored
75g packed fresh basil leaves
½ cucumber

225ml water
200g ice
Optional: birch xylitol or pure stevia to taste, if you need more sweetness

Dry-blend the pumpkin seeds. Add the lemon, chia seeds, apple, basil, cucumber, water and ice. Blend until smooth. If you need more sweetness, you can add a few drops of pure stevia or birch xylitol.

D-BURN TEA

Serves 15 (1 serving =1 cup)

10 teaspoons ground cinnamon

1 12.5cm piece fresh ginger, peeled and cut into chunks

10 peppermint tea bags

10 licorice tea bags

6 tablespoons flaxseeds

4.5 Litres water

Combine all ingredients in a pot. Bring the tea to a boil and then let it steep for 10 to 15 minutes. Strain and refrigerate for up to five days.

D-BURN SOUP

Serves 10 (1 serving = 450g)

Even after the plan is over, this soup is an excellent way to soothe your digestive tract.

2.25 Litres water

1.7kg chopped cauliflower

3 large spring onions, white and green parts, chopped

300g chopped green beans (trim the ends off if you prefer)

125g chopped asparagus, tough ends trimmed

160g chopped fresh coriander or parsley

2 garlic cloves, diced

1 dried bay leaf

1 green bell pepper, diced

1 to 2 jalapeño peppers, cored and diced

1 460g tin organic tomatoes (diced or whole)

1 carton vegetable broth, organic non-dairy

½ head celery, sliced

½ head red cabbage, chopped

2 tablespoons coconut aminos or tamari

½ teaspoon dried oregano

½ teaspoon dried rosemary

¼ teaspoon dried thyme

2 tablespoons sea salt

Combine all ingredients except the salt in a large pot over medium heat and bring to a boil. Reduce the heat to low, cover and simmer for 2 hours. Add salt during the last 5 or 10 minutes of cooking. Serve hot, warm or at room temperature. Refrigerate for up to 3 days. Freeze the remainder in individual serving sizes.

D-BURN LUNCH

LENTIL CHILLI

Serves 4

Although this recipe serves 4, you only actually need 2 servings—one for your Day 1 lunch and another for Day 4's lunch. Fortunately, this recipe freezes well, so set aside half for a future quick dinner for two after you are done with the D-Burn plan.

2 tablespoons extra-virgin olive oil or grapeseed oil
2 carrots, diced
1 red bell pepper, diced
1 celery stalk, diced
1 medium onion, diced
2 garlic cloves, diced
1½ tablespoons chilli powder
½ tablespoon ground cumin
½ tablespoon paprika
1 teaspoon dried oregano
¼ teaspoon cayenne pepper

¼ teaspoon freshly ground black pepper
1.5 Litres vegetable or chicken broth
200g dry lentils
1 425g tin black beans, drained and rinsed
1 425g tin diced tomatoes, with juice
½ teaspoon sea salt
75g sliced spring onion, white and green parts
40g chopped fresh coriander
Juice of 1 lime

Place a wide soup pot on the stove over medium heat. Place the oil, carrots, red bell pepper, celery and onion in the pot and cook, stirring often, for about 10 minutes, until the vegetables are nearly tender and beginning to brown. Add the garlic, chilli powder, cumin, paprika, oregano, cayenne pepper and black pepper. Sauté for 1 minute, then add the broth, scraping any browned bits from the bottom of the pan. Stir in the lentils and bring to a boil. Reduce the heat, cover and simmer for 30 minutes, or until the lentils are tender. Stir in the black beans, tomatoes and salt. Simmer for 10 minutes, then add the spring onion, coriander and lime juice. Serve.

D-BURN DINNERS

BEEF AND BROCCOLI BOWL

Serves 4

4 garlic cloves, diced

2 tablespoons diced fresh ginger

2 tablespoons tamari

2 tablespoons rice vinegar

½ teaspoon crushed red pepper flakes

450g sirloin or strip steak, sliced 6mm thick across the grain

4 tablespoons grapeseed oil

½ medium red onion, sliced

½ red bell pepper, cored, seeded and sliced

1kg broccoli florets

75ml beef or chicken broth

2 tablespoons sesame seeds

350g cooked quinoa

In a medium bowl, stir together the garlic, ginger, tamari, vinegar and red pepper flakes. Add the steak, stirring to coat, and set aside to marinate. Have ingredients ready by the stove, along with a large bowl.

Place a large, heavy frying pan with a lid over high heat. Heat 1 tablespoon of the grapeseed oil in the pan. Lift the beef out of the marinade (reserving the marinade) and add the beef to the pan. Stir-fry for 1 minute, just until the beef is no longer pink on the outside. Scrape the contents of the pan into the large bowl. Add another tablespoon of grapeseed oil to the pan, along with the onion. Stir-fry for 1 minute. Add the bell pepper, stir-fry for 1 minute more, then transfer the onion and bell pepper to the bowl.

Add the remaining grapeseed oil to the pan, then the broccoli and stir-fry for 1 minute. Add the broth, cover tightly and steam for 1 minute. Put the beef and veggies back in the pan, along with any accumulated juices, the reserved marinade and the sesame seeds, and stir until bubbling and heated through, about 5 to 10 minutes. Serve over quinoa.

SHEPHERD'S PIE

Serves 4

FOR THE TOPPING:

4 medium sweet potatoes, scrubbed
3 tablespoons raw coconut oil
½ teaspoon sea salt
½ teaspoon ground cinnamon
¼ teaspoon ground nutmeg
⅛ teaspoon cayenne pepper

FOR THE FILLING:

1 tablespoon extra-virgin olive oil
   or grapeseed oil
2 large carrots, diced
2 celery stalks, diced
1 medium onion, diced
1 teaspoon sea salt
2 garlic cloves, diced
¾ teaspoon ground chipotle
   pepper
½ teaspoon dried oregano
½ teaspoon ground cumin
¼ teaspoon ground cinnamon
450g minced turkey
240ml chicken broth

Preheat the oven to 220°C/425°F. Halve the sweet potatoes lengthwise and place them cut side down on a foil-lined baking sheet. Bake for 30 minutes or until tender. Set the sweet potatoes aside to cool.

While the sweet potatoes bake and cool, make the filling: heat a wide, deep pan or pot over medium-high heat. Place the oil, carrots, celery, onion and a pinch of salt in the pot and cook, stirring often, until the veggies are soft and starting to brown, about 10 minutes. Add the garlic, chipotle pepper, oregano, cumin and cinnamon, and sauté for 1 minute. Add the minced turkey and cook, stirring, until the meat is browned. Stir in the chicken broth, bring to a fast simmer, and cook for about 10 minutes, until the sauce thickens. Season with 1 teaspoon salt.

Meanwhile, when the sweet potatoes are cool enough to handle, scoop out the flesh with a spoon. In a food processor (or by hand), mash the sweet potato with the coconut oil, salt, cinnamon, nutmeg and cayenne pepper until smooth.

Spread the turkey mixture evenly in an 20 × 25cm baking dish. Spread the sweet potatoes evenly on top. Bake at 220°C/425°F for 15 minutes, and then grill for 1 to 2 minutes to brown the sweet potatoes around the edges.

STUFFED COURGETTES
Serves 4

4 medium courgettes (about 23cm long)
2 tablespoons extra-virgin olive oil
½ medium onion, finely chopped
½ red bell pepper, finely chopped
3 garlic cloves, diced
2 teaspoons ground cumin
1½ teaspoons sea salt

¼ teaspoon crushed red pepper flakes
450g lean minced beef
110ml chicken broth
175g cooked quinoa
40g chopped fresh mint
40g finely chopped fresh parsley

Preheat the oven to 190°C/375°F. Halve the courgettes lengthwise and then scoop out the seeds with a melon baller or sharp spoon, leaving about 6mm of flesh. Arrange the courgette shells snugly in a 23 × 33cm baking dish or on a rimmed baking pan.

Heat a large pan over medium-high heat. Place the oil, onion and bell pepper in the pan and sauté for 3 minutes. Add the garlic, cumin, salt and red pepper flakes and sauté for 1 minute. Add the minced beef and cook, stirring often, until browned, about 10 minutes. Add the chicken broth and scrape up any browned bits from the bottom of the pan. Raise the heat and simmer for 1 to 2 minutes, until the liquid has nearly evaporated. Remove from the heat and stir in the quinoa, mint and parsley.

Divide the filling among the courgettes, packing it tightly and mounding it up. Cover tightly with foil and bake for 40 minutes, until the courgettes are tender.

FENNEL AND SALMON

Serves 2

Note: this recipe serves only 2 because you don't need any leftovers, and it doesn't freeze very well.

4 garlic cloves, diced

2 tablespoons extra-virgin olive oil

2 tablespoons chopped fresh rosemary

1 teaspoon sea salt

¼ teaspoon freshly ground black pepper

2 medium fennel bulbs, sliced 12mm thick

½ medium red onion, sliced 12mm thick

1 red bell pepper, cored, seeded and sliced 12mm thick

2 175g salmon fillets

½ lemon

Preheat the oven to 230°C/450°F. In a large bowl, combine the garlic, oil, rosemary, salt and pepper. Scoop out 1 tablespoon of this mixture and set it aside. Toss the fennel, onion and bell pepper with the remaining oil mixture and spread evenly on a rimmed baking sheet. Bake for 20 minutes. Flip the veggies. Lay the salmon fillets on top, skin side down, and spread them with the 1 tablespoon of oil mixture that was previously set aside. Squeeze the lemon over everything. Bake for 10 to 12 minutes more, until the fillets are nearly opaque in the middle, and serve.

ITALIAN WONDER

Serves 2

Note: this recipe serves only 2 because you don't need any leftovers. If you are dining on your own, stash half in the freezer.

2 tablespoons extra-virgin olive oil
150g diced red onion
350g diced courgettes
250g diced yellow squash
150g sliced shiitake mushrooms
1 teaspoon sea salt
¼ teaspoon freshly ground black pepper
400g cherry tomatoes
1 garlic clove, diced
1 tablespoon chopped fresh rosemary
1 teaspoon dried oregano
110ml vegetable or chicken broth
1 tablespoon fresh lemon juice
75g pine nuts
2 tablespoons chopped fresh parsley
Optional: 175g cooked quinoa or wild rice

Heat a large frying pan over medium-high heat. Place the oil and onion in the pan and cook, stirring often, for about 4 minutes, until the onion begins to soften and brown. Add the courgettes, squash, mushrooms, salt and pepper. Cook for another 4 minutes, stirring often. Add the tomatoes, garlic, rosemary and oregano, and sauté for 4 minutes more. Stir in the broth and lemon juice, and scrape up any browned bits from the bottom of the pan. Simmer for 1 minute, until the sauce thickens. Stir in the pine nuts and parsley. Remove from the heat and season with salt and pepper to taste. Serve over quinoa or wild rice, if you like, or just enjoy it as is.

H-BURN RECIPES

On the H-Burn plan, the smoothie recipe serves 1 because you will make it fresh every morning. The tea and soup recipes make enough for the entire 10 days, but 10 days is a long time to leave tea and soup sitting in the fridge, so I suggest freezing half and defrosting it halfway through the week. Every lunch recipe serves 1 (double it if you are sharing) and every dinner recipe serves 2, but you will need to save half for a future lunch or dinner. If you need more than 1 serving for dinner, double or triple the recipe. The only exception is the Greek-Style Baked Cod, which also serves 2, but does not require saving half for later in the plan. Enjoy it with someone special.

H-BURN SMOOTHIE
Serves 1

40g raw sunflower seeds
450g fresh spinach
225g kale
1 whole grapefruit, peeled (if you are on statin drugs, use 1 whole orange instead)

¼ raw beetroot, peeled
1 tablespoon coconut oil
110ml water (or more, depending on texture and preference)
50g ice

Dry-blend the sunflower seeds. Add the rest of the ingredients to the blender and blend until the smoothie has reached your desired consistency.

H-BURN TEA
Serves 15 (1 serving = 1 cup)

6 organic limes, halved
7 milk thistle tea bags
7 dandelion root tea bags

1 tablespoon turmeric
4.25 Litres water (some will boil off)

Squeeze the limes into a large pot, then add the lime rinds and all other ingredients. Bring to a boil for 2 to 5 minutes, then let it steep uncovered for 1 hour. Cool, strain out the limes and tea bags, and store in the refrigerator. If you don't have enough room in your fridge, store half in the freezer and defrost it midway through the plan.

H-BURN SOUP
Serves 20 (225g soup + 225ml water = 1 serving)

Makes 10 servings, but note that this soup makes a concentrate, so when you prepare to eat it, dilute it with an equal part of water (so that in total, this recipe makes enough for 20 servings of soup). And remember, you can always make more—this is a free food!

1.7 Litres water
9 celery stalks, roughly chopped
900g chopped green beans
6 garlic cloves, smashed
9 courgettes, diced

330g button mushrooms
75g parsley
1½ onions, coarsely chopped
Sea salt to taste

Place the water, celery, green beans and garlic in a stockpot and cook for 5 minutes. Add the courgettes, mushrooms, parsley and onions, and cook for another 5 to 7 minutes, until tender. Let cool and purée in a blender, or blend in the pot with an immersion blender. When serving, dilute this concentrate with an equal amount of water, then heat and enjoy.

H-BURN LUNCHES

HERBED EGG SALAD

Serves 1

2 hard-boiled eggs, chopped

75g diced celery

1 tablespoon chopped spring onion, white and green parts

1 tablespoon finely chopped fresh parsley

1 tablespoon hummus

1 tablespoon Dijon mustard

½ tablespoon fresh thyme leaves

Sea salt and freshly ground black pepper to taste

150g torn romaine lettuce

150g thinly sliced fennel bulb

40g sliced fresh white mushrooms

1 tablespoon extra-virgin olive oil

1 teaspoon balsamic vinegar

175g pomegranate seeds (or serve with a fruit)

In a small bowl, combine the eggs, celery, spring onion, parsley, hummus, mustard, thyme, salt and pepper. Mix well. In a large serving bowl, toss the romaine, fennel and mushrooms with the oil and vinegar. Add more salt and pepper to taste. Top the lettuce mixture first with the egg salad and then the pomegranate seeds (or serve with a fruit).

CHICKEN AVOCADO SALAD WITH
CREAMY COCONUT-MANGO DRESSING

Serves 1

You could make extra chicken when prepping Day 1's dinner to use in this recipe (check out the recipe for Pan-'fried' Chicken with Fennel and Walnuts on page 244, and note that the amounts of chicken differ depending on whether you want to do this). If you don't, just cook your chicken fresh for this quick lunch.

110g boneless, skinless chicken breast
Sea salt and freshly ground black pepper to taste
1 teaspoon extra-virgin olive oil
450g fresh baby spinach
225g watercress
¼ avocado, sliced

FOR THE DRESSING:

1 mango, diced, with juices (or 150g thawed frozen chunks, diced; peaches or nectarines would work, too)
2 tablespoons coconut milk
1 tablespoon chopped fresh mint
2 teaspoons fresh lime juice
⅛ teaspoon lime zest
¼ teaspoon grated fresh ginger
⅛ teaspoon sea salt
⅛ teaspoon freshly ground black pepper
Pinch of crushed red pepper flakes

If you are not using leftover chicken from Day 1, place the chicken breast in a zip-top bag (or between two sheets of plastic wrap) on a cutting board. Pound it to a fairly even 8.5mm thickness and season generously on both sides with salt and black pepper. Heat a large non-stick frying pan over medium-high heat. Place the oil and chicken in the pan and cook the chicken until cooked through, about 4 minutes per side. Remove the chicken from the pan and set it aside to rest. In a large serving bowl, combine the mango, coconut milk, mint, lime juice, lime zest, ginger, salt, black pepper and red pepper flakes. Slice the chicken and add it to the dressing, along with the spinach and watercress. Toss to coat evenly. Season with salt and black pepper to taste, and top with the sliced avocado.

TUNA ROMAINE SALAD

Serves 1

1 175g tin water-packed tuna, drained

55g finely diced celery

40g finely diced spring onion, white and green parts

3 tablespoons hummus

1 tablespoon plus ½ teaspoon fresh lemon juice

Sea salt and freshly ground black pepper to taste

½ tablespoon extra-virgin olive oil

150g torn romaine lettuce

75g sliced white mushrooms

2 tablespoons chopped fresh basil

1 orange, segmented

2 tablespoons raw pine nuts

In a small bowl, combine the tuna, celery, spring onion, hummus, 1 tablespoon of the lemon juice, salt and pepper. Mix well. In a serving bowl, whisk together the oil and the remaining ½ teaspoon lemon juice. Add the romaine, mushrooms and 1 tablespoon of the basil to the dressing. Season with salt and pepper to taste. Top with the tuna salad, orange segments, pine nuts and the remaining 1 tablespoon basil.

NORI ROLLS

Serves 1

1 orange
1 tablespoon chopped fresh mint
1 teaspoon fresh lime juice
1 teaspoon tamari
¼ teaspoon grated fresh ginger
Pinch of crushed red pepper flakes
110 to 175g precooked small
  shrimp/prawns, shelled

200g thinly sliced Savoy or regular
  cabbage
4 nori sheets
4 asparagus stalks, tough ends
  trimmed
¼ avocado, sliced into 4 pieces
2 tablespoons sunflower seeds

Segment and dice the orange, saving the juice. In a large bowl, whisk together the orange chunks and their juice with the mint, lime juice, tamari, ginger and red pepper flakes. Add the shrimp/prawns and cabbage, and toss to coat.

Lay a nori sheet down and place one quarter of the filling on one side, leaving any excess liquid behind in the bowl. Top with one quarter of the asparagus, avocado and sunflower seeds. Starting with the bottom corner below the filling, roll the nori around the filling in an ice cream cone shape. Seal the edges of the rolls with a little bit of the dressing. Repeat for all four nori sheets.

SAVOY, WATERCRESS AND POMEGRANATE SALAD

Serves 1

150g sliced Savoy or regular
  cabbage
50g sliced celery
2 tablespoons sliced spring onion,
  white and green parts
85g hummus
Chopped fresh mint to taste

Sea salt and freshly ground black
  pepper, or tamari/coconut
  aminos, to taste
225g watercress or fresh spinach
175g pomegranate seeds
25g raw walnuts or sunflower seeds

In a large bowl, combine the cabbage, celery, spring onion, hummus, mint and salt and pepper. Mix well. Place the watercress on a plate and top with the cabbage mixture. Garnish with pomegranate seeds and walnuts.

H-BURN DINNERS

PAN-'FRIED' CHICKEN WITH FENNEL AND WALNUTS

Serves 2

This dinner serves 2, but make an extra 110g of chicken to use with Chicken Avocado Salad for your Day 3 lunch. Store it in an airtight container in the refrigerator.

225g boneless, skinless chicken breast

Sea salt and freshly ground black pepper to taste

1½ tablespoons extra-virgin olive oil

2 medium fennel bulbs, sliced 12mm thick

1 small onion, sliced 12mm thick

2 teaspoons dried oregano

2 garlic cloves, diced

240ml chicken broth

2 teaspoons balsamic vinegar

2 tablespoons chopped fresh basil

2 tablespoons crushed walnuts

Place the chicken in a zip-top bag (or between two sheets of plastic wrap) on a cutting board. Pound to a fairly even 8.5mm thickness and season generously on both sides with salt and pepper. Heat a large non-stick frying pan over medium-high heat. Place ½ tablespoon of the oil and the chicken in the pan and cook the chicken until cooked through, about 4 minutes per side. Remove the chicken from the pan and set it aside to rest.

Add the remaining 1 tablespoon oil to the hot pan. Then add the fennel, onion and oregano. Sauté for about 5 minutes, until the onion and fennel begin to caramelize. Add the garlic and sauté for 30 seconds more. Add the broth, bring to a boil and cook for about 5 minutes, until the broth has evaporated. Remove from the heat and stir in the vinegar. Add salt and pepper to taste. Slice the chicken and serve it over the veggies, sprinkled with basil and walnuts.

CORIANDER SHRIMP/PRAWNS AND GREEN BEANS

Serves 2

1 tablespoon coconut oil

175g green beans, trimmed and cut into 5cm pieces

1 small yellow squash, thinly sliced

1 small courgette, thinly sliced

350g raw shrimp/prawns, shelled and deveined

40g sliced spring onion, white and green parts

2 garlic cloves, diced

65ml coconut milk

1 tablespoon tamari

2 teaspoons lime juice

1 teaspoon grated fresh ginger

½ teaspoon lime zest

⅛ teaspoon crushed red pepper flakes

3 tablespoons chopped fresh coriander

Heat the coconut oil in a large, heavy frying pan over medium-high heat. Add the green beans and stir-fry for 1 minute. Add the squash and courgette and stir-fry for 2 minutes. Add the shrimp/prawns, spring onion and garlic, and stir-fry for about 1 minute more, until the shrimp/prawns turn pink. Add the coconut milk, tamari, lime juice, ginger, lime zest and red pepper flakes. Continue to stir for about 5 minutes, until the shrimp/prawns are cooked through and everything is hot. Remove from the heat and serve topped with the coriander.

ROASTED SPAGHETTI SQUASH WITH SHIITAKE MUSHROOMS
Serves 2

1 large spaghetti squash
2 tablespoons extra-virgin olive oil
Sea salt and freshly ground black
  pepper to taste
225g minced beef
110g sliced shiitake mushrooms
150g chopped onion
2 garlic cloves, diced

2 teaspoons chopped fresh
  rosemary
1 teaspoon dried oregano
240ml chicken broth
1 tablespoon tamari
3 tablespoons chopped fresh
  parsley

Preheat the oven to 205°C/400°F. Cut off the squash's stem end. Halve the squash lengthwise, scoop out the seeds (an ice cream scoop works great), and place the halves cut side up on a baking sheet. Brush them with ½ tablespoon of the oil and season generously with salt and pepper. Roast the squash for 40 minutes, or until you can easily scrape the strands out of the squash with a fork.

While the squash is roasting, make the sauce. Heat the remaining 1½ tablespoons oil in a large frying pan over medium-high heat. Add the minced beef, mushrooms, onion, garlic, rosemary and oregano, and sauté for about 5 minutes, until the beef is browned. Add the broth and tamari. Bring to a boil, then reduce the heat and simmer for about 8 minutes, until nearly all of the liquid evaporates.

When the squash is cool enough to handle, use a fork to scrape out all of the strands into a large bowl. Season the squash with salt and pepper. Top the spaghetti squash with the meat sauce and parsley.

ROASTED CAULIFLOWER AND SALMON

Serves 2

2 tablespoons extra-virgin olive oil

Juice and zest of ½ lemon, plus 2 lemon wedges for serving

2 garlic cloves, diced

3 tablespoons chopped fresh dill

Pinch of crushed red pepper flakes

¼ teaspoon sea salt

¼ teaspoon freshly ground black pepper

2 175g salmon fillets

1.3kg cauliflower florets

½ medium red onion, cut into 8 wedges

Prepared horseradish to taste, for serving

Preheat the oven to 230°C/450°F. In a small bowl, combine the oil, lemon juice and zest, garlic, 2 tablespoons of the dill, red pepper flakes, salt and pepper. Brush the fish generously with about half this mixture and set it aside on a plate. Toss the cauliflower and onion with the remaining half of the oil mixture and spread it on a baking sheet. Roast the vegetables for 15 minutes. Stir the veggies and then place the salmon on top, skin side down. Bake for 12 to 15 minutes more, or until the fillets are nearly opaque in the middle. Season again with salt and pepper; top with the remaining 1 tablespoon dill. Serve with horseradish and lemon wedges.

STUFFED CABBAGE ROLLS WITH WILD MUSHROOM SAUCE

Serves 2

You need only six large cabbage leaves for this recipe, but you can use the remaining cabbage for the Savoy, Watercress and Pomegranate Salad on page 243.

FOR THE CABBAGE ROLLS:

1½ teaspoons extra-virgin olive oil

100g finely chopped onion

50g finely chopped celery

2 garlic cloves, diced

½ tablespoon minced fresh rosemary

½ tablespoon fresh thyme leaves

Sea salt and freshly ground black pepper to taste

225g minced beef

2 tablespoons raw pine nuts

6 large Savoy or Napa cabbage leaves

240ml chicken broth

FOR THE SAUCE:

1 tablespoon extra-virgin olive oil

225g wild or crimini (baby bella) mushrooms, sliced

¼ teaspoon sea salt

¼ teaspoon freshly ground black pepper

1 garlic clove, diced

120ml chicken broth

1 tablespoon fresh thyme leaves

1 teaspoon fresh lemon juice

1 teaspoon tamari

2 tablespoons chopped fresh parsley

Preheat the oven to 175°C/350°F and set a large pot of salted water to boil. Heat a large non-stick frying pan over medium heat. Place 1½ teaspoons oil and the onion, celery, garlic, rosemary, thyme and a pinch of salt and pepper in the pan and sauté for about 5 minutes, until the onion and celery are tender, and then set the mixture aside in a large bowl. When it has cooled a bit, mix in the minced beef, pine nuts, ¼ teaspoon salt and ¼ teaspoon pepper.

Add the cabbage leaves to the boiling water and blanch them for about 5 minutes, until they're pliable. Remove the leaves gently with tongs. Lay the leaves out flat and cut out the thickest part of the centre vein, to make them easier to roll.

Divide the beef mixture evenly among the 6 blanched cabbage leaves. Fold in the sides and roll up. Place the rolls seam side down in a 20cm square baking dish. Add 240ml broth to the pan, cover loosely with foil and bake for 1 hour.

When the cabbage rolls are nearly done, make the sauce. Heat a frying pan over medium heat. Place 1 tablespoon oil and the mushrooms, salt and pepper in the pan and sauté for about 5 minutes, until the mushrooms release their liquid. Add the garlic and sauté for 30 seconds more. Add the broth, thyme, lemon juice and tamari. Simmer until the liquid is nearly evaporated, about 4 minutes. Serve the cabbage rolls with a spoonful or two of their broth and top with the mushroom sauce and parsley.

ROSEMARY CHICKEN WITH ROASTED VEGGIES
Serves 2

225g fresh beetroots, trimmed
2 small yellow squash
2 celery stalks
1 small sweet onion
Juice of ½ lemon
2 garlic cloves, chopped
2 tablespoons grainy mustard

2 tablespoons extra-virgin olive oil
1½ tablespoons chopped fresh
   rosemary
¼ teaspoon sea salt
¼ teaspoon freshly ground black
   pepper
2 bone-in, skin-on chicken thighs

Preheat the oven to 230°C/450°F. Cut the beetroots, squash, celery and onion into 4cm chunks. In a large bowl, combine the lemon juice, garlic, mustard, oil, rosemary, salt and pepper. Add the chicken thighs to the bowl, turning them to coat both sides, and then set them aside on a plate. Add the chopped vegetables to the bowl and toss to coat. Spread the vegetables evenly in a 23 × 33cm baking dish. Bake uncovered for 10 minutes. Add the chicken (skin side up) and bake uncovered for another 40 minutes, or until the chicken is browned and cooked through and the vegetables are tender.

VEGGIE QUICHE

Serves 2

2 large leeks, white and light green parts, thinly sliced
1 tablespoon extra-virgin olive oil
75g sliced shiitake mushrooms
125g sliced asparagus, tough ends trimmed, sliced diagonally into 5cm pieces

450g fresh spinach
2 teaspoons fresh thyme leaves
Sea salt and freshly ground black pepper to taste
4 large eggs
90ml coconut milk
2 tablespoons chopped fresh basil

Preheat the oven to 175°C/350°F. Rinse the sliced leeks thoroughly to remove any grit and drain well. Heat the oil in a large frying pan over medium heat. Sauté the leeks and mushrooms for about 5 minutes, until the mushrooms have given up their liquid. Add the asparagus and sauté for 4 minutes more, or until the leeks are nearly tender. Add the spinach and thyme. Stir for about 1 minute, until the spinach wilts. Remove the pan from the heat, season with a pinch of salt and a crack or two of pepper, and set aside to cool a bit.

In a large bowl, whisk together the eggs and coconut milk, another pinch of salt and a few cracks of pepper. Stir in the veggie mixture. Pour into a 23cm pie plate and bake for 30 minutes, or until the quiche is golden brown and puffed and the centre is set. Let the quiche rest for 5 minutes before slicing. Sprinkle with the basil.

GREEK-STYLE BAKED COD WITH ARTICHOKES

Serves 2

1 tablespoon extra-virgin olive oil
½ medium red onion, cut into 8
  wedges
300g sliced courgettes
250g sliced yellow squash
1 garlic clove, diced
2 teaspoons fresh thyme leaves
Pinch of sea salt

Freshly ground black pepper to
  taste
1 400g tin artichoke hearts, drained
  and quartered
8 kalamata olives, chopped
Juice and zest of ½ lemon
2 175g cod fillets
1 tablespoon chopped fresh parsley

Preheat the oven to 230°C/450°F. Heat a large ovenproof frying pan over medium-high heat. Add the oil and sauté the onion, courgettes, squash, garlic, thyme and a generous pinch of salt for about 5 minutes, until the veggies are crisp-tender. Remove from the heat and stir in the artichoke hearts, olives, and lemon juice and zest. Season the cod fillets with salt and pepper and nestle them in the vegetable mixture. Bake uncovered for about 15 minutes, until the cod is nearly opaque in the centre. Sprinkle with parsley and serve.

CHAPTER TEN

Living Your Life on Fire

So you've incinerated your plateau, broken through your weight loss resistance and the scale is moving again. Maybe your swelling is down and you can see your cheekbones and natural ankles again. Maybe your belly is flatter; what were lumps are now curves. You're cinching your belt a notch or two tighter, or you're back into your skinny jeans. Maybe you finally have that body you want.

Now what?

You've taken your remedy, your medicine in the form of food. You have healed the problem for now, and you are ready to live your life again. Or maybe getting you unstuck in one area of your body has unveiled another layer of much-needed repair. Either way, it's time to get back on your weight loss path, or nurture your newly tweaked metabolism, integrating what you now know into a whole-body approach to healthy eating.

After *The Burn*, I'm not going to leave you hanging. Life is complex and the body is complex and there is always more to do. It's time to take a look at where you are, so I can help you to move forward into your best life. Ask yourself:

- Do you have more weight to lose, and now that the scale is moving again, you're ready to burn it up?

- Did you fix one issue but want to tackle another one? Maybe your swelling has come down and now you're ready to attack that spare tyre.

- Are you right where you want to be and you want to make sure you stay there, without the weight creeping back on or your shape morphing back into something you don't like?

- Now that you are on the road to health and off the road to chronic disease, are you motivated to keep your energy high and your health strong?

- Do you tend to swell, or get IBS symptoms, or have chronic PMS and you want to keep those issues under control?

- Are you worried you will fall back into some of your old bad habits?

- Will you miss some of your favourite parts of *The Burn*?

This chapter is about what to do next. *The Burn* is not a lifestyle. I don't suggest my clients eat like the meal plans on *The Burn* every day for the rest of their lives, because *The Burn* uses foods at a therapeutic level to evoke change. If you were to stay on the I-Burn, the D-Burn or the H-Burn for months at a time, that would be like taking antibiotics forever. You've pulled out the splinter and now you're ready to move on. After you pull out a splinter, you don't keep going at it with the tweezers. You turn your attention to other things and use those tweezers for something else, like your eyebrows.

But do not forget about the amazing and powerful tools you have at your disposal. Continue to use them both preventively and therapeutically. Your body will tell you what you need, if only you will listen. The body whispers, then it talks, then it yells, then it screams. Listen and look for subtle cues that inflammation is elevating, or your digestion is off, or your hormones feel out of balance.

Your body told you that you needed the I-, D- or H-Burn, and what you do next depends on where you are now. There are so many ways to use elements of *The Burn*, as well as my other programmes, to get to your goals and maintain your weight, health and energy. This is your road map.

DO YOU HAVE MORE WEIGHT TO LOSE?

The Burn set you back on track to lose the weight you weren't losing. It kick-started your weight loss and incinerated your plateau. But now that you're unstuck, what's the best longer-term weight loss plan?

If you need to lose weight and the scale is moving down again, hear me now: go immediately to *The Fast Metabolism Diet*! If you're new to the FMD world, welcome. If you're already one of my existing "virtual clients", then hello, my friend! When I have a client who breaks through a plateau but still needs to lose more weight, I immediately put her or him on a 28-day cycle of the FMD. I believe this is the right road map for weight loss for almost anyone because it is a thorough and complete metabolism repair programme. FMD consists of 28 days that you can do once to lose about twenty pounds, or more than once if you have more to lose. Once you are unstuck, you need to repair a broken metabolism and this is a great way to do that. You must rehabilitate your broken metabolism.

I strongly suggest you read *The Fast Metabolism Diet* because there is important information to achieve total repair. Each food and each recipe is hand-selected to evoke the correct macronutrient levels for the specific phase, to evoke healing of each system in each phase. All the food lists, the recipes and the *whys* are in the book.

CAN YOU REPEAT *THE BURN*?

Yes. If you were super stuck and you feel like you are making progress but you haven't quite shaken loose as fully as you would like, you can do your *Burn* plan again. I typically don't recommend doing this for more than three cycles, however. That's nine days on the I-Burn, fifteen days on the D-Burn or thirty days on the H-Burn. This is fine if you really want to keep up with those plans and intensely focus on one area. However, after three cycles, you can get in a different sort of rut and it's time to shake it up again, with either another *Burn* plan or *The Fast Metabolism Diet*. Remember: if anything you are doing that was working for you *stops working*, then that's a sign that you aren't giving your metabolism enough variety. You need to shake it up and try something different. Your body is telling you that it needs you to change something.

You cannot hurt yourself doing *The Burn* plans too many times. They are nourishing and complete. It's just that they don't have as much variety as other plans, and after three cycles you won't get the same bang out of them as you were getting before. If you do take a break, you can always go back to the plan you love in a few weeks or months and it will work again.

This is why the FMD is so effective—it changes what you are doing three times every week. You can stay on it longer and enjoy continued results. But like anything else, if that stops working then try something new yet again. Go back on *The Burn*. Try a different plan. Whatever it is, keep it moving and changing to keep your metabolism fired up and the excess fat burning off.

HOW I USE *THE BURN* IN MY CLINIC

Here are a few scenarios that demonstrate how I use *The Burn* in my clinic:

1. A client selects the plan that is most fitting based on symptoms. They do it once, and then they go back to the *Fast Metabolism* lifestyle (what our virtual clients call Phase 4, or the maintenance phase of FMD) because they are at a healthy weight.

2. They do the *Burn* plan that most closely addresses why they are stuck, in order to break through a weight loss plateau. Then they go on the FMD to continue their weight loss.

3. They are significantly stuck and they identify strongly with one area. They are in need of a more prolonged and intense repair, so they stay on their particular plan for three consecutive cycles. Then, if they need to lose more weight, they go on the FMD, or if they have reached their ideal weight, they transition to the *Fast Metabolism* lifestyle.

4. They have a long history of health and weight issues and identify with issues on all three of the *Burn* plans. In this case, I have them

work through all the plans, doing the I-Burn, then the D-Burn, then the H-Burn, then repeating that cycle several times in order to rotate between intense repairing of all three systems. I will keep them on this rotation as long as they continue to lose weight. If the weight loss slows, then I move them to the FMD.

Once you've got *The Burn* as well as the FMD under your belt, you have access to five different and powerful strategies: the I-Burn, the D-Burn, the H-Burn, the FMD and the *Fast Metabolism* lifestyle. This is a solid and significant amount of information you have now. And these are just five of the many plans I have in my own toolbox! I will continue to introduce these to you in future books and other media, but with these five options alone, any individual can set up a successful system for health that can last a lifetime. (If you are a health coach, you can use any of these approaches in your own programme as well. I have a training programme for nutritionists and health coaches for how to use these strategies with clients—check my website for information, if you are interested.)

SHOULD YOU TRY A DIFFERENT *BURN* PLAN NEXT?

If, like many of my clients, you have symptoms and issues related to all three of the plans, and you have done the plan that addressed your most pressing issues, you can then go back and do a different plan. Maybe GI distress was bothering you the most, but now your stomach feels calm and looks much flatter. Hooray! But maybe you would still like to tackle those swollen ankles and puffy cheeks, or now you're noticing that pesky little PMS week that you dread and wondering if you can fix it. Just break out the I-Burn or the H-Burn next, and see what that does for you. You can do all three plans in a row (and then do them again) and get all your systems working better.

ARE YOU READY FOR MAINTENANCE?

Maybe you just had a little bit to lose. Maybe it wasn't about the weight, but more about how your body was distributing your weight or the symptoms that were plaguing you. Maybe no matter what your weight, you couldn't get rid of your cellulite, or your belly, or your digestive symptoms. Clients come to me fine with the number on the scale, but they want to get rid of the lumps on their thighs or the roll around their midsections. Maybe you just felt weird or "off", and your body wasn't looking or feeling right to you. Now, after *The Burn*, everything is where it should be and you feel great.

What do you do now? This is the time to find a place to "live", and fall in love with food and all it can do for you. I want my clients to live a healthy life with sound nutrition. I do believe you should be on a diet for the rest of your life. But remember, for me, diet means D.I.E.T.: Did I Eat Today?

Did I eat to repair my metabolism?

Did I eat to reduce inflammation?

Did I eat to halt fat storage?

Did I eat to scavenge subcutaneous fat, yellow fat and/or white fat?

Did I eat to heal and shrink my gut?

Did I eat to achieve hormone balance?

Did I eat to nourish my thyroid, reverse diabetes and/or increase my libido?

Once you've done *The Burn*, you don't have to leave it all behind. You can continue to use the parts of the plans you liked the best. The first time you do the plan, you need to do it exactly as I've laid it out, and do it all the way, so your body receives the intense repair it needs. After that, maybe you don't need to do a ten-day H-Burn. Maybe you just need to break out the H-Burn Tea for a few days to get over a hormonal hump. Maybe you just need to start your day with an I-Burn Smoothie to depuff your face. Maybe the D-Burn Soup is just the remedy for a twitchy stomach. Maybe you loved the I-Burn Tea or the H-Burn Soup or the D-Burn Smoothie. You can keep the things you loved in your regular rotation because they will always be therapeutic. There is nothing wrong with doing *part* of *The Burn* on most days, or whenever you feel the need.

I also encourage you to live by a few basic rules that I always recommend:

- Eat five times every day to keep your metabolism fired up. That's three meals and two snacks every day. For a biodiverse micro- and phytonutrient-rich grocery list, combine all the foods from the three phases of this plan.

- Eat every three to four hours (except when you are sleeping!). This helps stabilize blood sugar and keeps cortisol balanced, digestion moving, fat converting to fuel and your body converting food into life.

- Eat within thirty minutes of waking every day. This is so important for your autonomic nervous system balance as well as for getting your metabolism fired up right at the beginning of the day, for maximum burn. Drink half your body weight in ounces of water every day. Remember, dilution is the solution for pollution . . . and toxins cause inflammation, poor digestion and hormone dysfunction.

- Eat organic whenever possible. The higher up the food chain, the more important this is. Dairy, eggs, poultry and meat are worth the investment in organic and hormone-free.

- Avoid meats cured with nitrites and nitrates. These preservatives halt rancidity in food by slowing the breakdown of fat. Ingest these and you will slow the breaking down of your own fat.

On most days, I suggest a rhythm like this for my clients who are not working on a specific health issue or symptom:

BREAKFAST	1 serving each: Fruit Veggie Protein Grain
SNACK	1 serving each: Veggie Healthy fat with protein, i.e., whole egg, raw nuts, hummus, salmon

LUNCH	1 serving each:
	Fruit
	Veggie
	Protein
	Healthy oil

SNACK	1 serving each:
	Veggie
	Healthy fat with protein, i.e., whole egg, raw nuts, hummus, salmon

DINNER	1 serving each:
	Veggie
	Protein
	Healthy oil
	Optional: Grain

One thing to note is that you might want to experiment with how well you handle grains at dinner. Do grains make you calm or tired? Full of energy? Bloated? Try eating them less or more, depending on how your body and you do. Don't eat anything your body has a negative response to, no matter how "healthy" someone tells you it is. I once had a client who had chronic stomach aches, rashes on the back of her arms and dark circles under her eyes, but was off all of the common food allergens. After working together, we found out she was allergic to apples, broccoli and strawberries. These were all the things she was told to eat because they were so healthy. Don't tell your body how it should be feeling. Listen to how it *is* feeling.

I recommend staying away from these metabolism-killing foods *most* of the time:

Wheat

Corn

Dairy

Soy

Refined sugar

Caffeine

Alcohol

Dried fruit

Fruit juice

Artificial sweetener

Fat-free "diet" foods

As a rule, we try to keep these things outside our house. Then we don't have to worry so much if they find their way into our food on our adventures. The exception: diet, fat-free, artificial sugar foods are *never* OK in my world.

If you really need some caffeine or corn chips or ice cream or a margarita, go ahead and indulge if they happen to fall into your mouth. Remember, garbage burns when your metabolism is a roaring fire, but make sure to eat well on a regular basis to keep your metabolism on fire.

There will likely be many times in the future, throughout your life, when you will find you need to break out *The Burn* again. You might go on antibiotics, or slip in your eating habits and start retaining fluid, or find yourself in the throes of menopause, or be in a chronic overwhelming stress situation. You might contract a virus or have significant toxicity exposure or suddenly notice you've taken on some cellulite or hard belly fat or fluffy white fat in a new place. Life happens. You've got these tools in your toolbox for a reason, so let's look at what can happen that can justify breaking them out again.

ARE YOU STUCK, BUT IT'S DIFFERENT THIS TIME?

So there you are, living and feeling great, making good decisions—and suddenly you start to gain weight again. Or maybe you've been losing at a steady clip since you did *The Burn*, but suddenly you hit another plateau.

This is very common, and most often I find that a new plateau or a new period of weight gain isn't necessarily caused by the same things as the last plateau or period of weight gain. Life changes and you are always changing, too. This is why I've given you three plans. What works for you today might not be what is right for you tomorrow, and after you thought everything was going great, sometimes something else goes wrong.

I had a client who had been stuck at a plateau for a long time. She had a lot of inflammation and she also had Hashimoto's disease, which is an autoimmune disorder. Because Hashimoto's involves a strong inflammatory response, I put her on the I-Burn, and when her weight started to move again, I put her on the FMD for two cycles. She lost 35 pounds, but then she got stuck again. She was having a lot of constipation, so we interjected with the D-Burn. This got her unstuck again. All her medical tests were improving and she was feeling great, but then she got stuck again. This time, her periods were scanty and she was having spotting between cycles. So you guessed it—I put her on the H-Burn. When she got unstuck, she went right back to FMD again, and I'm happy to report that she has now lost over 120 pounds!

This isn't uncommon with my clients who have a lot of weight to lose. It's like peeling away layers of an onion—or layers of subcutaneous, white or yellow fat. They are often able to use all three *Burn* plans at different times during their weight loss journey, but as they need them. The body is an incredible and multilayered organism, and the life we live is diverse and multidimensional.

Sometimes you're doing just great, and then something completely unexpected happens to stall you or throw your progress into reverse. A client of mine was at her ideal body weight, give or take a couple of pounds. She ate well and exercised regularly. Then she had an injury and had to take some steroid medication. Suddenly, her inflammatory markers were through the roof. Because of the steroids, her adrenals were wiped out and she felt both wired and tired. We polished her off with the I-Burn and she was able to get right back on track. It took several I-Burn cycles because her inflammation was so severe, but by the time she was done rehabbing her injury, we had rehabbed her metabolism.

Another client I hadn't seen in years had lost about 34 pounds on FMD and was maintaining beautifully. Then one day while scuba diving, she was scratched by some coral and got a staph infection. She had to go on three weeks of IV antibiotics. This completely trashed her digestion, killing off the healthy, good microflora. She gained only six pounds, but she had significant bloat as well as alternating constipation and diarrhoea. When she called me, I put her immediately on the D-Burn, and within five days she was feeling amazing.

You never know what's going to happen. You might first read this book and discover you desperately need the D-Burn, and it's a flaming success. Other issues may be completely off your radar. Maybe the idea of menopause doesn't even ring a bell in your world. You don't relate to that at all. But two years down the line, suddenly you're in the throes of perimenopausal symptoms and you're developing that hard fat that you're finding is impossible to get off. Now you've got the tools to deal with that—the H-Burn is here for you.

You need to continually monitor and listen to what your body is telling you so you know the right course of action. When you are on a roll, you don't need to be unstuck. Stay the course. But when you hit a wall, you have to do more for your body, and not necessarily ask more from your body. We've all heard "exercise more and eat less". This is just crazy because food is what promotes weight loss, and too much hard exercise is a stressor for the body and can promote weight gain— but this is exactly the cuckoo philosophy prescribed by so many in the diet world. Not only does this not work, but it can have exactly the opposite effect. I can't tell you how many starvation-diet, hard-exercisers I've seen in my clinic who are stuck and can't lose a pound. We have to look at the *whys*. Why aren't you losing? And what is your body telling you to do?

The more you can identify with the *whys*, the more specific you can be, the better you will understand what to do. Maybe the D-Burn worked before because you were having digestive or respiratory issues, but now those are resolved. What's going wrong this time? Is it hormonal? Is it inflammatory? Look inside and listen. The most important thing I want you to take away from this book is that when you get stuck, do not just keep doing more or less of the same thing you've already been doing. That is never the answer to breaking free of an impediment in life or in your diet. If you come across a boulder in your path, you don't just keep walking into it over and over, hoping it's going to go away. You have to do something different. You have to stop walking and start climbing, or change your course.

I want you to live your life most of the time in a way that will prevent you from getting stuck, but I know how life goes. Life happens, and these plans are all here for you when you need them. Your body is in a constant state of adaptation, so pay attention and you will know exactly what to do. Listen to your body and give it what it's asking for; it will tell you what it needs. Look at where you are stuck and pull the trigger on one of these plans.

HOW DO YOU RECOVER FROM OVERINDULGING?

I'm realistic. It's always good to know you're going to "go there", or admit that you've been overdoing it. These are the times when I like to prescribe a controlled *Burn*. For example, you go on vacation, you go to a party, you have a girls' night out or a special date, or it's the holidays. Food is celebratory and there are many occasions in life to celebrate.

Let's say you know you'll be going out to a Brazilian restaurant full of heavy meats and comfort foods. Knowing you might have some digestive issues afterward, you can schedule a D-Burn starting the next day—the best programme for post-indulgence recovery. Or drink your D-Burn Tea the day before and the day of, to prepare your body for a gut-busting event.

I have a client who often travels to New York, and whenever she does, she gets constipated, so she takes digestive enzymes and probiotics, and we always plan a D-Burn for her when she gets home. She used to take laxatives, but then it took weeks for her to get straightened back out. Now she just pulls out the D-Burn and she feels great, no medication required.

When it comes to a night of drinking, the I-Burn is your best friend. Alcohol, preservatives and additives stimulate inflammation. Colourful fruity drinks, such as those margaritas from the machine or those pink neon drinks, are the worst for inflammation. Maybe you have a night out on the town planned. You know you're going to party like a rock star. But you can decide ahead of time to recover afterward with the I-Burn. Or, just break out the I-Burn when you wake up the next morning with a headache and a swollen face and ankles. Even if you just brew some I-Burn Tea while you blow-dry your hair, your body will handle your night out much better.

Then there's the classic PMS binge. If you know you get raging PMS during the second half of your cycle and you're going to eat everything in sight, preferably covered in chocolate, then preemptively strike with the H-Burn, to calm and minimize your symptoms as well as help with recovery after you've had a hormonal-based overindulgence. You might just find that you won't have that three- to five-pound weight gain this time around—and you might not need quite so much chocolate, either. If you're already PMS-ing—how often do you forget it's coming and then suddenly find yourself snapping at someone and ravaging the cabinets for chocolate?—then get on the H-Burn stat. When the hormones become imbalanced, the body craves sugar, sugar and more sugar. Even if it's just a little bit of candy, you'll still need a lot of the H-Burn Soup. It will make a big difference in how you come out on the other side next week.

IS THERE A REASON TO DO *THE BURN* EVEN WHEN I FEEL GREAT?

The Burn is absolutely suited for prevention. All three of the plans in this book are designed to nurture, enhance, enrich and support you, so although your dramatic intervention is over, I want you to understand how to use your new knowledge to refine your results and prevent future roadblocks from inhibiting your progress and your life.

In nature, a systematic burn supports the flow of life. In a forest, lightning strikes and creates a fire, and that enriches the soil to support nutrients and growth. It's the same thing with *The Burn*. You can use it to follow the natural cycles in your body. Few things in our environment push us toward health on a daily basis. If you eat, drink, sleep, live, you will be exposed to things that encourage the slow march toward disease. Doing *The Burn* preventively is a phenomenal way to counteract this, gently encouraging your body toward health.

If you do the plans on a regular basis, such as once a year or twice a year, or once a season, or even once a month, you can stay ahead of any problems. Call on *The Burn* at the slightest hint of an issue. When you notice your ankles are swollen, intervene with the I-Burn. When you notice an unpleasant rumble in your stomach, call in the D-Burn forces. When you know you're going to have PMS next week, nip it in the bud with the H-Burn.

But you can also continue to do *The Burn* on a regular basis even before you show any symptoms. Try a plan you haven't tried yet. If you did the I-Burn, try the D-Burn. If you did the H-Burn, try the I-Burn. These plans are always therapeutic for anyone, anytime.

One thing I like to suggest to my clients is to do the plans on a schedule, such as quarterly, or in sync with the seasons, or even every other month. This is a great way to use *The Burn* preventively. In the spring, when allergies are common, do a preventive I-Burn and you may barely experience a sneeze. In the autumn, when root vegetables are in season, do a preventive D-Burn to really turn up the heat so you can successfully digest those veggies and heavier winter foods to come. Combat the winter blues with a preventive H-Burn as soon as the days start to get shorter and the weather gets chilly.

Some of my clients rotate through the three soups for prevention. I have a history of eczema and food allergies, to the point of anaphylaxis and EpiPens. I find that my body craves the I-Burn Tea when it is reactive (which is most of the time). I know that when I've got a lot on my plate and I'm crazy busy, I should make a ginormous batch of I-Burn Tea and sip on it all day long.

YOUR BODY TELLS YOU WHAT IT NEEDS

The bottom line is that it's your *Burn*. Use it however your body needs it. What all of these situations and scenarios boil down to is that your body tells you what it needs. When you learn your body's language, then it won't be a mystery which plan you need or what you need to do when things get off track with your weight loss, your health or your general well-being. The more you work with the *Burn* plans, the more you will discover that there are times when the recipes on the D-Burn plan, for example, sound just amazing. They make your mouth water. At other times, your eyes might stray to those I-Burn foods. Pay attention to this. It isn't random.

Again, your body is always speaking to you, and living your life on fire is about listening. Your body speaks through mild discomforts and symptoms that are easy to ignore but are whispering messages to you nevertheless. It speaks through your cravings, which are calls for something you need, and it speaks to you through your energy level. When you feel energetic, you are doing something right, and when you are low on energy, your body is crying out to you for something it needs. If you are feeling blue or depressed, your body is saying, "I need the H-Burn!" If you are having a bad time with allergies, your body is murmuring, "How about a little I-Burn?" If your stomach starts acting up after a weekend of overindulgence, your body is quietly pleading: "Let's do that D-Burn again! Please?"

I have a seventeen-year-old client who has been diagnosed with polycystic ovarian syndrome (PCOS), and she always craves the H-Burn Soup. I feel good on the H-Burn Soup, but she *needs* it. Her mom makes her batches and batches, and it has become a staple in their house. Sometimes she adds prawns or meatballs to the soup to make it an entire meal. If you look at the ingredients for the H-Burn Soup, it doesn't exactly look like something a teenager would go wild for, but she listens to her body, and her body tells her what she needs. I've told you about how I crave the I-Burn Tea when my life gets crazy because it helps with the inflammation related to my personal health issues. I can't tell you how many calls and e-mails I get from clients asking for the one thing they remember helped them the most: "Remember that one soup you made after I had to take those antibiotics and I got all gassy and bloated and looked like I was six months pregnant? Can I have some more of that?" "Remember when my skin broke out and I was retaining water and you gave me that smoothie recipe?" "Remember when I had that bout of IBS and that one tea made me feel so much better?" "Remember when I was having a hard time with perimenopause and you made me that one soup? Can you send me the recipe?"

You have two ears and one mouth for a good reason. You should be listening twice as much as you speak, and listening to your body twice as much as you are telling it what you think it should be doing for you. We say some pretty terrible things to our bodies, things we would never say to anyone else. We tell our bodies they look fat, or have big thighs, or jiggle too much, or sag, or wrinkle, or disappoint us. Blah, blah, blah. Your body is doing the best it can with the environment you provide, and when it needs something more, it tells you—it tells you by collecting body fat, by swelling, by bloating, by jiggling and sagging and wrinkling. Enough with the finger-pointing. Instead, listen. Listen, listen, listen. Stop telling it what's wrong and start listening to what it's asking for.

Another fantastic thing about *The Burn* is that it not only teaches you to listen to your body, but it teaches your body to speak up. Your body isn't always aware of what you are missing until you expose it to that missing element and your body lets out a big sigh of relief: *Ahhh, that's exactly what I need!* Once you expose your body to what it needs, it will start to ask for more because now it knows those things are available. Listening will get easier because the message is coming through more clearly.

But if you aren't listening, you won't hear. Whether your body is whispering, talking, yelling or screaming, or whether the symptoms associated with the I-Burn, D-Burn or H-Burn plan are profound or mild or barely there, each of these plans can prevent your issues and every one of them will intensify and polish your glow. Each one does it differently, but they all do it. They are here for you, so use them, use them, use them.

Finally, remember that food is medicine and it is powerful. You can resolve many if not most chronic physical issues by targeting them with the right foods. This book shows you three powerful ways to do this. They are serious power tools, but they are just three of the many tools I have to offer you.

So consider this: when you need 28 days of total body metabolic repair, *The Fast Metabolism Diet* is there for you. When you hit a plateau or are stuck and want to target a very specific result, *The Burn* is here for you. If you want community support, new recipes and inspiration, my website, newsletter, blog posts and social media are here for you. In short, *I am here for you*, and I plan on us having a long and fruitful relationship.

We have come far together on our journey, and I want to continue to peel back the layers for you, to show you the many amazing and miraculous ways you can use food as medicine. There are many exciting and therapeutic ways that you can turn to nature to fix the *why* and heal what's wrong. This will build you into the most radiant, healthy, strong, energetic, beautiful, fit and resilient version of yourself. I have plenty more tricks in my bag to show you, and so many more gifts to give you.

Let's keep our sleeves rolled up and continue to sculpt your body, mind and spirit with the power of food.
Bon appétit!

Haylie

ACKNOWLEDGEMENTS

There will never be enough ways to thank my incredible literary agent, Alex Glass. He has been my advocate and champion far beyond the literary arena. Tina Constable, you can inspire and light a fire with such grace and conviction that you make me believe in myself and my vision. Heather Jackson, my fierce editor, thank you for moulding the clay and pushing me to give our community more with each book without ever editing me out of a single page.

Eve Adamson, only with your mad skills could I have pulled this off. How can you be so professional and such a dear friend? I thank you for getting me and my voice, and taking my clinic to my virtual clients. Chris Frietchen, you have watched this brand and community like a mother hen and have cherished what is valuable to me as if it was your own. This is a special thank-you to you from me: you never judged, you just shared the vision and made sure in my times of weakness or insanity that we never veered. Melanie, who keeps me focused on the purpose for doing all of this and the holistic map of my journey, I thank you from the bottom of my heart. I am so fortunate to work with the world's best publisher and for the incredible people on my team: Maya Mavjee, Aaron Wehner, Diana Baroni, Meredith McGinnis and Tammy Blake; thank you for getting this into the hands that it can help the most.

Bob Marty, my partner in creating a special for public television, I thank you for making one of my lifelong dreams come true. You are so talented; I am in awe of you.

I want to give a heartfelt thank-you to our active and supportive community; your dedication to the movement and compassion for others inspires me each and every day. Grassroots do indeed grow strong. I want to give a call out to the independent Facebook groups that have formed as a result of individuals sharing their struggles and successes, as well as their passions and desire to help others. I am honoured to have you all in my world. A special shout out to the FMD Support Group, the FMD IT GRUPPO DI SUPPORTO and the Fast Metabolism Diet Group.

And to my amazing clients who have been very patient and flexible through this whole process. You all know you have a special place in my heart and I thank you so much for allowing me to be on your journey to health. I learn so much from you; thousands of lives are being changed because of it.

And then there is my team. Kym, Leilani, Keyanna and John, if you only knew how much your support means to me and the hundreds of thousands of lives you and your efforts have touched. The world is a better place because you all are in it.

Thank you to the Weins family, who gave me three majestic weeks to connect with my family, nature, newfound friends and bears.

To my beautiful family, whose patience and encouragement through this all has been lifesaving, I love you more than you will ever know and I thank you so very much. To my stud of a husband, my angelic kids, my mom and dad, my sisters, my aunt and grandmother, and my nieces and nephews, the book is done. Dinner is at my house!

There are countless individuals that have helped manifest this project, I thank you all!

INDEX

Italian Wonder, 236
shiitake, health benefits, 147
Shiitake, Roasted Spaghetti
    Squash with, 246
Tuna Romaine Salad, 241
Veggie Quiche, 250
Wild, Sauce, Stuffed Cabbage Rolls
    with, 248–49

N
Neem oil, 190–91
Nori Rolls, 242
Nostril breathing, alternate, 203–4
Nuts. *See also* Pine nuts; Walnuts
    soaking, 193–94

O
Oil pulling, 191
Olive leaf extract, 192
Omega-3 fatty acids, 155
Oral health, 191
Oranges
    Nori Rolls, 242
    Tuna Romaine Salad, 241
Overindulging, 263–64
Ozone therapy, 220

P
Parsley
    compounds in, 72–73
    H-Burn Soup, 238
    I-Burn Tea, 223
Pau d'arco
    for detox bath, 186–87
    health benefits, 182, 186
    tea, 182–83
Pectin powder, 212
Peppercorns, black, 205
Peppers
    Fennel and Salmon, 235
    Lentil Chilli, 231
Perimenopause, 55
Phlegm, 43, 46

Physical issues
    general symptoms, 21
    paying attention to, 265–67
    remedied by D-Burn Plan,
        39–40
    remedied by H-Burn Plan, 51–53
    remedied by I-Burn Plan, 28–29
Phytonutrients, 149
Pine nuts
    Hummus Coleslaw, 226
    Italian Wonder, 236
    Roasted Vegetables on Courgette
        "Pasta", 227
PMS (premenstrual syndrome),
    263–64
Polycystic ovarian syndrome
    (PCOS), 55–56
Pomegranate
    health benefits, 212–13
    Herbed Egg Salad, 239
    Savoy and Watercress Salad,
        243
Portion guidelines, 70
Prawns. *See also* Shrimp
Probiotics, 185
Protein
    on the D-Burn food list, 116
    on the D-Burn grocery list, 95
    on the H-Burn food list, 161
    on the H-Burn grocery list, 124
    on the I-Burn food list, 88
    on the I-Burn grocery list, 71
    serving sizes, 70
Psyllium fibre, 213
Puffiness, 21
Pumpkin seeds
    D-Burn Smoothie, 229

Q
Quiche, Veggie, 250
Quinoa
    Beef and Broccoli Bowl, 232
    Stuffed Courgettes, 234

ABOUT THE AUTHOR

HAYLIE POMROY has spent more than twenty years helping people lose weight, overcome health challenges and reach their ideal health while still enjoying real food and not going hungry. She's the author of two *New York Times* #1 bestsellers: *The Fast Metabolism Diet* and *The Fast Metabolism Diet Cookbook*.

With integrative health care clinics in Burbank and Fort Collins, Haylie is highly regarded in Hollywood and the medical community. She provides collaborative care with physicians from institutions such as the Children's Hospital of Orange County, Children's Hospital Colorado, the UCLA Medical Center, and Brigham and Women's Hospital (Boston). Her impressive client list includes celebrities such as Jennifer Lopez, LL Cool J, Cher, Raquel Welch and Robert Downey, Jr. Haylie discovered her guiding philosophy, "food as medicine", after helping hundreds of clients—famous and not—improve and manage their health issues.

Haylie received her B.S. degree in animal science from Colorado State University. She then turned to human health, becoming a Registered Wellness Consultant in 1995, specializing in holistic health, nutrition, exercise and stress management. She received her level II certifications from IABP in Fort Collins, Colorado, where she went on to sit as the director of the academy for four years.

She received advanced certifications from the Institute of Quantum and Molecular Medicine in EDS, Health and Wellness Principles, Homotoxicology, Autotoxic Therapies, Biological Terrain, Heart Rate Variability and Noncognitive Biofeedback. She is also a certified Holistic Health Counselor.

She has appeared on *The Dr Oz Show*, *Good Morning America*, *Katie*, *Extra* and *Access Hollywood*, and has been featured in *First for Women*, *People*, *Harper's Bazaar*, *Marie Claire*, *New Beauty* and more.

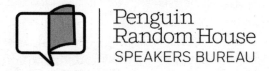

Penguin
Random House
SPEAKERS BUREAU

To inquire about booking Haylie Pomroy for a speaking engagement,
please contact the Penguin Random House Speakers Bureau at
speakers@penguinrandomhouse.com. A full profile and video footage
of Haylie Pomroy can be found at www.prhspeakers.com.

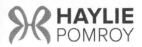
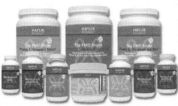
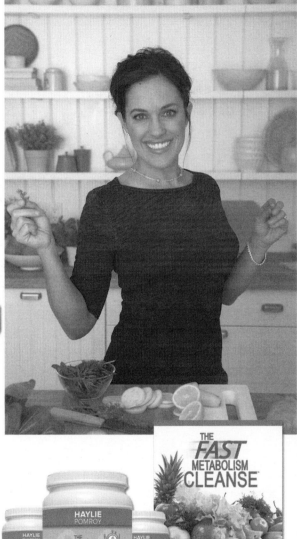